T0131251

The Eczema Diet

'My family members have had great success on *The Eczema Diet* and I believe it will be a valuable and powerful tool for improving the general health and the skin of millions of eczema sufferers around the world. I highly recommend it to all families with allergic and atopic conditions to improve their health and wellbeing. It uses some simple principles that highlight the importance of healthy living, food and nutrition to alter our immune system and prevent and treat allergic and immunological conditions like eczema.'

Dr Gary M. Leong, MBBS, FRACP, PhD

The Eczema Diet

Eczema-safe food to stop the itch
and prevent eczema for life

Karen Fischer

BHSc, Dip. Nut.

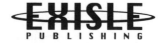
EXISLE
PUBLISHING

This edition published in 2014

First published in 2012

Exisle Publishing Pty Ltd
'Moonrising', Narone Creek Road, Wollombi, NSW 2325, Australia
P.O. Box 60–490, Titirangi, Auckland 0642, New Zealand
www.exislepublishing.com

Copyright © 2012 & 2014 in text: Karen Fischer

Karen Fischer asserts the moral right to be identified as the author of
this work.

All rights reserved. Except for short extracts for the purpose of review,
no part of this book may be reproduced, stored in a retrieval system
or transmitted in any form or by any means, whether electronic,
mechanical, photocopying, recording or otherwise, without prior
written permission from the publisher.

A CiP record for this book is available from the
National Library of Australia.

ISBN 978 1 921966 46 0

Initial design concept by saso content + design
Design and typesetting for this edition by Tracey Gibbs
Typeset in Minion Pro
Printed in Shenzhen, China, by Ink Asia

This book uses paper sourced under ISO 14001 guidelines from well-
managed forests and other controlled sources.

10

Disclaimer
This book is a general guide only and should never be a substitute for
the skill, knowledge and experience of a qualified medical professional
dealing with the facts, circumstances and symptoms of a particular
case. The information presented in this book is based on the research,
training and professional experience of the author, and is true and
complete to the best of their knowledge. However, this book is
intended only as an informative guide; it is not intended to replace
or countermand the advice given by the reader's personal medical
team. Because each person and situation is unique, the author and
the publisher urge the reader to check with a qualified healthcare
professional before using any procedure where there is a question as
to its appropriateness. The author, publisher and their distributors are
not responsible for any adverse effects or consequences, loss, claim or
action that may arise from reliance on the information contained in
this book. It is the responsibility of the reader to consult a qualified
healthcare professional regarding their personal care. This book
contains references to products that may not be available everywhere.
The intent of the information provided is to be helpful; however, there
is no guarantee of results associated with the information provided.

KAREN FISCHER is a nutritionist and a member of the Australian Traditional-Medicine Society (ATMS). She has a Bachelor of Health Science Degree (BHSc) from the University of New England and a nutrition diploma (Dip. Nut.). In 2008, Karen's bestselling book *The Healthy Skin Diet* won 'Best Health, Nutrition or Specific Diet Book' at the prestigious Australian Food Media Awards. In private practice, Karen's patients are almost exclusively babies, children and adults suffering with eczema. For more than a decade, Karen has used the Eczema Diet to help her patients become eczema-free. Karen is frequently a guest nutritionist on Australian television and has written health articles for Australian, New Zealand and UK publications.

Karen's other books with Exisle Publishing include:
The Healthy Skin Diet
Healthy Family, Happy Family, and
Younger Skin in 28 Days.

For more information on all of these titles please visit:
www.exislepublishing.com

Contents

Introduction

My daughter Ayva was two weeks old when she developed spots on her face that resembled acne. The creases of her elbows and knees were red and weeping, and she would often scratch until her arms bled. When she was ten months old, a nurse from the local Early Childhood Centre, who had seen Ayva a few months earlier, exclaimed, 'Has your child *still* got eczema?' I thought what a rude comment, eczema is a genetic condition and *what could I do about it*? I was a nutritionist and I had not considered looking at treatment options for my baby beyond cortisone cream and thick ointments.

When Ayva was one she was diagnosed with dust mite allergy, which meant she could no longer sleep with, or touch, any of her soft toys. We were advised to avoid junk food, additives and salicylates. Playing on the grass, swimming in a pool and patting the family cat inflamed Ayva's skin from head to toe so the cat was sent to grandma's house and swimming lessons were cancelled. Then one day Ayva, who was growing resentful about being different from her friends, ate some food at a friend's birthday party and her eczema spread further down her legs. We noticed she was becoming more sensitive to everything and it was sad to see her suffering.

I began researching eczema. By the time Ayva was two I had devised a basic diet and supplement routine for her, and two months later, to my surprise and excitement, her eczema was gone. The temporary dietary changes were strict but soon Ayva could enjoy normal activities such as playing with fluffy toys, swimming in chlorinated pools and occasionally she could eat party food without her eczema returning, and she no longer needed topical steroids. Her diet was gradually expanded and eventually she could eat all foods without her eczema returning.

Research shows that eczema sufferers spend up to $2000 on eczema treatments each year and 36 per cent of sufferers spend more than 10 minutes each day applying topical steroids and emollients. Despite this, the number of people with eczema is rising and has *tripled* in recent years. Now *20 per cent* of people in the developed world have eczema and it's mostly babies and children who are suffering.[1]

- One in five children suffers from eczema.
- There are more than 6 million eczema sufferers in the United Kingdom, and 31.6 million people have eczema in the United States.
- There are 1 million eczema sufferers in Australia and almost 6 million Australians will suffer from eczema at some point in their life.
- In New Zealand, more than 10 per cent of people have eczema.

The eczema statistics may continue to rise if we do not address the main factor that determines our genetic health: our diets. According to Ordovas and Corella from the Nutrition and Genomics Laboratory, Jean Mayer–U.S. Department of Agriculture: *Food intake is the environmental factor to which we are all exposed permanently from conception to death. Therefore, dietary habits are the most important environmental factor modulating gene expression during one's life span.*[2] While it is okay to use modern medicines to help you or your child gain temporary relief, a long-term solution usually involves dietary changes.

My daughter is now twelve years old and the Eczema Diet has changed a lot since I first devised this program. For the past ten years, my eczema patients have been giving feedback about the program, which enabled me to refine the Eczema Diet. One of the things I love most about my job is reading research papers on skin health. I'm often in my home office until well past midnight, reading medical documents published on eczema, even ones dating back to the 1800s (a dangerous time to have eczema as doctors often prescribed toxic heavy metals which occasionally caused fatalities!). In the late 1800s, some hospital-based doctors advocated dietary changes, which were effective in eradicating eczema. By the mid 1900s, topical steroids became popular and diet research slowed during this time. However, in the last 30 years nutrition research for eczema has increased in popularity. *The Eczema Diet*, particularly chapters 2, 3 and 6, presents this research in detail.

However, if you or your child are suffering and keen to get started, it's fine to skip the first few chapters and begin at Chapter 4 'The Eczema Diet: how it works'. Then as you follow the program you can read chapters 1 to 3 and do the handy questionnaires in Chapter 2. If you have a baby with eczema, this research and the questionnaires are still relevant to you as you can use them to analyse your family diet before conception and the dietary information becomes practical once your baby starts eating solids.

What is the Eczema Diet?

At first glance the Eczema Diet may seem like a regular elimination diet but it differs in many ways. The Eczema Diet is designed *specifically* for eczema sufferers. While on the Eczema Diet, you *temporarily* take problematic foods out of the diet and you eat nutritious 'eczema-safe' foods that strengthen the health of your entire body. The Eczema Diet is incredibly nutritious and as your (or your child's) eczema clears up, a wider variety of foods are reintroduced to the diet so you can enjoy most — if not all — foods and remain eczema free (if you have severe allergies continue to avoid your allergy foods until given clearance by your doctor). Once the skin barrier function is restored, dust mites are no longer a problem and you can resume normal activities such as swimming and playing with pets.

The Eczema Diet is presented in three parts. Part 1 is all about your skin and is rich with tips on how to manage and mend your eczema. Part 2 has useful non-diet information that you can refer to at any time if you need a bath recipe, moisturiser advice or a quick itch-busting treatment. And Part 3 contains the eczema-safe recipes, shopping guides, food charts and menus for each specific age group, from babies to adults, as well as a party food guide for special occasions. Please keep in mind you will need to tailor this advice to suit your individual allergies, health requirements and eczema, and there is separate advice for babies, children and adults.

I know that right now, while you have eczema, it can be painful, and incredibly itchy. And it can be heartbreaking to see your child or a close friend suffering. Sometimes your toughest challenges call you to find new and more effective solutions, and to take action and find what really works for you. I hope you enjoy the program and I wish you well in your endeavour to create beautiful, eczema-free skin.

Health and happiness,
Karen

The Eczema Diet has a facebook page and a monthly newsletter.
See www.facebook.com/TheEczemaDiet for more information

Medical note

Before beginning the Eczema Diet it is important to have your skin condition diagnosed by a GP or dermatologist. If you have any medical conditions that are being treated with diet or drugs, you should follow the Eczema Diet with the supervision of your doctor, nutritionist or dietician.

Note: When the term 'eczema' is used throughout this book, it also refers to dermatitis, unless otherwise stated.

Did you know?

Which famous screen goddess of the 1950s and '60s suffered for long periods with eczema throughout her childhood and as a teenager?

Brigitte Bardot

Success stories

'Georgia's skin condition has really started clearing up over the past four to five weeks. Georgia (Gigi) woke up a couple of days ago and said, "Mum, I don't have eczema any more!" She was so excited. She still has lots of scar tissue on her feet and on the back of her knees that I hope in time will fade, but all the redness, inflammation and soreness has gone … You are a true blessing Karen … I'm so excited! Life for us has never been better and I can thank you for most of that! Ever since Gigi was eight months old I have tried every doctor, dermatologists, naturopaths, Chinese medicine, dieticians, old wives remedies etc., and no one has explained eczema to me like you have. Your book is a bible and should have a place in everybody's home.' **Amanda Essex, Qld**

'The dietary changes and advice Karen gave us worked and two months later Jesse's eczema was gone. It's great, Jesse doesn't need medications anymore. I could finally throw away the Advantan® as we had found the source of the eczema rather than masking the symptoms. I liked the fact that the diet allowed us to find the specific foods he was reacting to, and it was very straightforward and easy to follow. Friends and family were amazed and asked how I got his skin looking so good.' **Linda, Minchinbury, NSW**

'My sixteen-month-old son Jagger has suffered with eczema since birth, especially on his feet and behind his knees. After I put him on Karen's anti-eczema program, within a couple of days he was sleeping better and scratching less. Within ten days all the redness was gone from his skin and I could leave him without clothes, and without scratching! He's much happier and busy playing instead of scratching!' **Karma Montagne**

'The diet plus all the supplements worked so well for us. I felt like a miracle happened to Leo. (He had regular steroid creams from a very early age, on top of antibiotics for infections on the skin that often happened because of various reasons, including childcare and very itchy nights …) We had flaxseed oil and probiotics and other natural supplements before, but I think the combination and diet that you described is the most effective. (I also learnt a lot for myself, for my own health! Many thanks for this too.) My younger one also has a bit of eczema, but just few spots, which is such a relief! When we did the diet, we had it pretty much for the whole family. Milan's eczema also completely disappeared.' **Natalya**

'I've had eczema since birth. A specialist diagnosed my condition as chronic eczema. My skin, especially my face and neck, hurt and itched constantly, I was always tired and often irritable; I'd accepted that it would be with me for life ... Thanks to Karen's program I am now clear of eczema (none, zilch, not a skerrick). The real turning point came when I started taking the eczema supplement Karen developed. My energy levels increased, I could finally kick the sugar and for the first time in my life I became eczema clear. I was amazed! To maintain really healthy skin I always start the day with Karen's smoothie. I now use a far lighter moisturiser and much less of it on my face and body. My family has even commented how they love Mummy's new soft skin. Thank you Karen, my only regret is that I didn't find your program sooner.' **Mary Washington**

'Hi Karen, I would firstly like to thank you so much for your help with my son's eczema. Not only does my son have his skin back, but he is so much more confident. You see, he is quite timid and having just started school this year was extremely paranoid about his "itchies". I was getting quite upset and stressed as nothing would work and we had tried so many things: skin specialists, three naturopaths, Bowen therapy, Australian Biologics, NAET therapy and even went back to his paediatrician. He had a swim program at school which he was very upset about attending as he would have to show his skin and some kids had already asked about it. As a result, he would go to school on hot days with a jumper on as he wanted to keep covered and when I told him he was to now wear his summer uniform to school he got so upset. It's heartbreaking when your little boy cries to you and asks you, "When will my itchies go away, Mum?" and you've exhausted every avenue and still have no answer! So on behalf of Jacob, I thank you so much for your fantastic book.' **Claudine Hardy**

'I have been recently trying your advice about giving my five-year-old, who suffers terribly from eczema, a daily dose of the supplement for salicylate sensitivity. I must say that after three days his skin is beautiful. I have never seen it look this good. Combined with your diet I am so grateful for a different child.' **Cathi Firth**

'My son Luca suffered from severe eczema as a baby. We saw you several times approximately three to four years ago for advice. My son is fully cured thanks to your help.' **Bronwyn Air**

'Dear Karen. My four-year-old daughter, who is about to start kindy, has been taken off preservatives and artificial colours and has been taking her supplements for her severe eczema and is looking like a million dollars. What a difference in just six weeks. After four years of battling her eczema (not sleeping, not eating, extreme fatigue and hospitalisation with infected skin) I am now in control, more than ever. The doctors told me it was all about maintaining her comfort. The Healthy Skin Diet maintenance program is sooooo much better than many, many tubes of cortisone cream that I used to use.' **Meaghan**

'Clare has gone from vomiting up to ten times a day to just once a week. She hasn't had any rashes for at least a fortnight. Clare stopped vomiting within three to four days after starting the diet and supplements. Her twin sister Reese is also a "new" baby girl … She's gone from a grumpy whinger to a happy little girl in the last few weeks. I am keeping the "new" baby! Reese's personality change happened about ten days to two weeks after starting the new diet.' **Jenny Bangor**

'After two weeks on the Eczema Diet I'm stunned by the good results and my wife is speechless (just strokes my eczema-free hands and then looks at me in disbelief). I never thought it could work this quick!' **Andrew McGlone**

'I have been itching non-stop for six months and have eczema on arms, legs and face and more widespread in winter. I have been praying hard for a solution. I got one with your book. Within three days I have no itch and my skin is clear. THANK YOU for writing *The Eczema Diet* — you are literally the answer to my prayers!' **Barbara**

'Hi Karen, I just wanted to give you an update on Darcy. His back, wrists, ankles and the insides of his arms have cleared up. I also wanted to say thank you from the bottom of my heart. You have changed me and helped to improve my son's happiness and life. Your work is amazing and what you have done for my family and others is just life-changing.' **Rhianna**

'I am happy to say that Komal is 99 per cent out of her eczema! Her skin is dry but all the rashes have gone. Your advice and diet chart has helped to bring down the severity. She has a happy diet and her skin is smoother. Her skin colour is also improving. Regards and thanks.' **Anandhi**

Eczema + diet

To appreciate the healing power of food you. must first have something to heal.

Chapter 1
Healthy skin + eczema

Your skin is not only something you hope (and pray) looks good as you step out of your front door each day; like your heart and lungs, your skin is a vital organ that keeps you alive. Your skin is a barrier and a filter between the outside world and your insides, which is why the outermost layer, the *stratum corneum*, is known as 'the skin barrier' (see Diagram 1). The skin barrier helps to protect your body from excessive water loss so you don't die from dehydration. It helps to regulate your body temperature so you don't 'cook' your internal organs and it protects you from invading microbes such as dust mites and bacteria. A normal skin barrier is thick and the outermost layers of dead skin cells flake off in a barely detectable manner, as the outermost binders snap and release the unwanted cells (see Diagram 2a on p. 12).

Diagram 1: Human skin

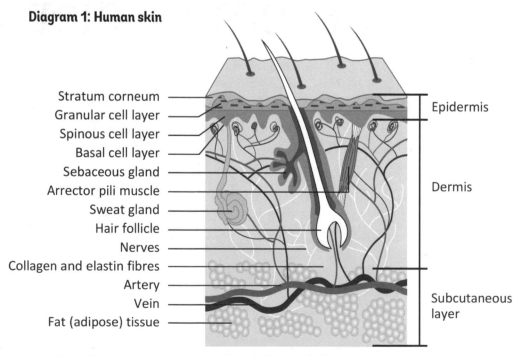

New skin cells form at the bottom of the epidermis and when they're ready they move towards the stratum corneum. In normal, healthy skin this trip takes about four weeks.

Eczema diagnosis

Eczema is generally diagnosed using the following criteria. Firstly, you *must have* itchy skin, plus three or more of the following symptoms:

- itchiness in the skin creases, such as the folds behind the knees and elbows, fronts of the ankles or around the neck (children under four years may also have it on their cheeks)
- dry skin
- visible eczema affecting the outer limbs, cheeks or forehead
- symptoms appearing within two years of birth (not always an indication, but very common)
- family history of asthma, hay fever or (if under four years old) a history of atopic disease in a first-degree relative.[1]

Know your lingo

Atopic: describes an allergy-prone individual and includes eczema, asthma and hay fever.

Dermatitis: any generalised inflammation of the skin.

Eczema: derived from a Greek word meaning 'to boil out'.

Skin barrier function

A useful way to describe the basic structural changes the skin goes through when you have eczema is demonstrated in the 'brick wall' model of the skin, which was created by professor Michael Cork and colleagues Danby and Hunter from the University of Sheffield in the United Kingdom. In this model, skin cells are likened to bricks which are held together by iron rods (binders called corneodesmosomes) and mortar (lipids, which are fats).[2]

When you have eczema, the skin barrier is usually thinner than normal so its protective capacity is compromised (see Diagram 2b on p. 12). The binders that hold the skin cells together in the deeper layers of the skin snap too early, causing premature flaking of the skin, and the fatty lipids in between your skin cells have cracks which appear throughout the skin barrier.[3]

Irritants, including soaps and detergents, enhance the snapping off process of the binders, the skin cells break down prematurely and deeper cracks appear in the skin (see Diagram 2c). As the skin barrier breaks down, the cracks allow allergens, such as dust mites and bacteria, to enter the skin (Diagram 2d).[4] This contributes to flare-ups and can lead to infections and immune responses, including allergic reactions.

Diagram 2: The brick wall analogy of the skin barrier

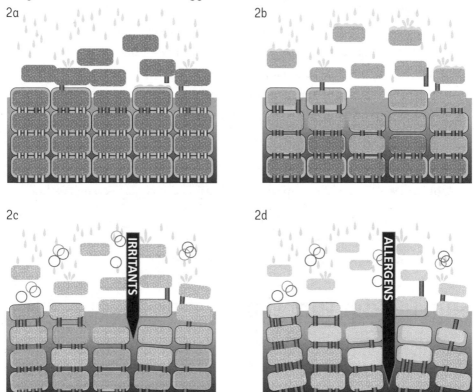

Diagram printed with permission from Cork and Hunter.

The acid mantle

With the exception of newborn babies (who have a skin pH of close to neutral), healthy skin has an acidic pH of approximately 5.5. This is known as the 'acid mantle'. The acid mantle protects the skin from harmful microbes, decreases the colonisation of 'free-loading' pathogenic bacteria and fungus, and promotes the adhesion to the skin of beneficial (non-pathogenic) bacteria. Research shows that eczema sufferers can have skin that is not acidic enough, making the skin barrier less protective and practically defenceless against microbes, such as dust mites and *Staphylococcus aureus.*[5] However, to improve the acid mantle of your skin so it's more resilient to dust mite invasion and weather extremes, you can take a calcium supplement. Calcium supplement information can be found on p. 117.

Historical eczema prescriptions

In *The British Medical Journal* back in 1882, a doctor described a diet that rapidly cured his eczema-afflicted patients. He documented a particularly 'hopeless case' of a nine-year-old boy who had suffered from eczema since he was five months old. The child had been under constant medical care, in and out of hospitals for more than eight years and no prescribed treatment, cream or drug had ever improved his eczema. When he was admitted to hospital for eczema treatment on this occasion, the doctor placed the child on a modified diet. The diet was low in fat, dairy-free and sugar-free. All fat was cut off meats, and poultry was recommended instead of pork. An oil supplement was prescribed. Beef broth was given, with the fat carefully skimmed off and he ate baked fish, not fried.

Within a fortnight the child's skin showed improvement and a month later his eczema was practically gone and he was discharged from hospital.[6]

Chapter 2

Eczema + diet: 60 years of research

Eczema is a unique skin disease with many factors associated with its appearance. The last 60 years of research offer some fascinating clues into how your diet (or the diet of your parents) can contribute to the appearance of eczema. While some aspects of eczema and genetic health cannot be explained, this chapter is devoted to the scientific research on how diet can affect eczema-related gene function and (most importantly) what you can do about it. Included in this chapter are eight factors associated with eczema (there are more factors discussed in chapters 3, 6 and 8). If you are not keen on reading the scientific information presented in Chapter 2, you can skip these paragraphs, if desired, and focus on the Recommendations, which are listed in dot points in shaded boxes, and the Questionnaires, which can help you to identify problem areas in your diet and health.

Genetic defects

Eczema is not contagious, so you can't catch it from someone if you touch their skin, but chances are you inherited it from your parents. If you have one parent with eczema, you have a 20 per cent risk of developing eczema yourself. If both parents suffer from eczema, hay fever or asthma, your chances of developing it jumps to between 50 and 80 per cent. According to the research, eczema is regulated by approximately four or five major genes; some affect the immune system while others weaken the skin barrier.[1] For example, all genes come in pairs and some eczema sufferers can have one or two defective copies of the filaggrin genes (the protein that binds keratin fibres in the epithelial cells in human tissue).[2] Approximately 10 per cent of the British population have a single defective copy, so they suffer from dry, flaking skin.[3]

Genetics and dietary factors

Your diet affects your genetic health in a variety of ways. In the *American Journal of Clinical Nutrition*, Professor Loren Cordain and her colleagues say that our dietary changes, which began with the introduction of agriculture and animal farming about ten thousand years ago, may have occurred too recently for our human genetics to adapt.[4]

There are various problems with today's diets, which include the following:

- The glycaemic load has increased. Processed foods usually have a higher glycaemic index (GI), which elevates blood glucose and insulin levels.
- We consume the wrong ratios of fats: our diets are low in omega-3 fatty acids and rich in saturated fat, and processed vegetable oils and margarines cause the overconsumption of omega-6.
- We have fewer micronutrients in our diet. Processed foods often contain sugar and white flour, which are low in vitamins and minerals. Deficiency in just a single nutrient can cause genetic defects that can lead to the appearance of eczema.[5]
- The acid–alkaline balance has been altered. Western diets can cause low-grade metabolic acidosis that worsens with age.
- The sodium–potassium ratio has altered. There has been a 400 per cent increase in salt ingestion, while potassium-rich fruit and vegetable consumption has plummeted.
- Fibre content has decreased. Refined sugars, vegetable oils, alcohol and dairy products are devoid of fibre, and refined grains contain much less fibre than wholegrains.[6,7]

Over the last 200 years, food manufacturers have introduced highly processed foods containing artificial colours, preservatives, sweeteners and flavour enhancers. Our biological make-up hasn't had enough time to become accustomed to this barrage of artificial additives.[8] According to the Food Intolerance Network in Australia, in 2009 there were 1154 food products containing problematic colour additives in Australia and in the United Kingdom there were more than 1000 products containing problematic food colourings that can worsen eczema symptoms and cause a range of side effects. And population studies confirm that acne and eczema are rare in traditional cultures where processed foods are not a regular part of the diet.[9,10]

Your genes can be modified by your diet

As mentioned in the introduction, American researchers claim that our dietary habits are the most important environmental factor modulating gene expression during one's life span.'[11] According to German researchers, essential fatty acids in the diet can modify gene expression, T-cell function, cell membrane fluidity and cell signalling.[12] In experimental studies, dietary carotenoids modulate gene activity to protect against inflammatory damage and tumour growth.[13] And in one of the largest gene–diet interaction studies ever conducted, involving analysis of more than 27,000 people from five ethic groups (European, South Asian, Chinese, Latin American and Arab), the effect of diet on genetic health was confirmed yet again. Researchers reported that a healthy diet rich in raw vegetables and fruit modified the gene variants located on chromosome 9p21, which is the strongest marker for heart disease. A healthy diet significantly weakened this gene's damaging effects.[14]

Your diet greatly affects your genetic health, and this chapter covers the research and the dietary ways to improve your genetic health and ultimately prevent eczema.

Allergies

An allergy is an abnormal immune response triggered by a normally harmless substance. In eczema sufferers, allergic reactions can cause a worsening of eczema symptoms, coughing, sneezing, wheezing and, in severe instances, anaphylaxis (a difficulty in breathing caused by a life-threatening swelling of the tongue and/or throat). Allergic reactions can be measured as allergy sufferers have raised levels of immunoglobulin E (IgE), the antibody found in your blood and tissues that mediates allergy. Allergy tests include the skin prick test, measuring serum-specific IgE, and for children under the age of three there is a skin application food test. IgE-dependent, food-allergic reactions cause a sharp rise in the blood histamine level (this is a vital piece of information) and histamine toxicity occurs, which causes the negative symptoms you experience when you're having an allergic reaction.[15,16,17]

Histamine toxicity and diet solutions are covered shortly.

Table 1: Common food allergies associated with eczema

Common food allergies in eczema sufferers	Percentage with allergy
egg (hen's)	71
peanut	65
dairy products, cow's milk	38
other nuts	34
sesame seeds	18
wheat	13
soy	4

Allergy tests are useful but keep in mind they only identify a limited number of possible food allergies and even if you've been allergy tested you may still be exposing yourself to foods you are sensitive to. Do the following questionnaire to see if you have food or environmental allergy symptoms.

Questionnaire 1: Allergy symptoms

Circle any symptom/s you experience on a regular basis, then circle the corresponding answer (YES / SOMETIMES / NO) that best describes the frequency of that symptom or collection of symptoms. YES = weekly or daily; SOMETIMES = monthly or occasionally; NO = never or rarely.

1. **Nasal symptoms. Do you have …**
   - ❀ itchy nose
   - ❀ sneezing
   - ❀ wheezing
   - ❀ nasal drip
   - ❀ blocked or 'stuffy' nose
   - ❀ and/or a crease at the end of the nose from frequent rubbing/itching/ wiping of drips

   YES / SOMETIMES / NO

2. **Skin symptoms. Do you have ...**

- ❀ hives
- ❀ skin rash
- ❀ itchy skin
- ❀ eczema
- ❀ facial flushing
- ❀ rosacea
- ❀ acne
- ❀ foul or abnormal body odour
- ❀ excess perspiration
- ❀ and/or swelling (lips, tongue, eyes, throat ...)

    YES / SOMETIMES / NO

    Note: If you experience swelling, see your doctor or go to a hospital as you may be having an anaphylactic reaction.

3. **Eye symptoms. Do you have ...**

- ❀ dark rings under the eyes (allergic shiners)
- ❀ puffy eyes
- ❀ itchy eyes
- ❀ conjunctivitis
- ❀ eye pain and/or
- ❀ temporary blurred vision

    YES / SOMETIMES / NO

4. **Gastrointestinal symptoms. Do you have ...**

- ❀ diarrhoea
- ❀ constipation
- ❀ colic
- ❀ excessive or smelly gas
- ❀ indigestion
- ❀ gastrointestinal bleeding
- ❀ nausea
- ❀ stomach or abdominal cramps/pains
- ❀ vomiting
- ❀ bad breath

❋ loss of appetite

❋ and/or acid reflux

YES / SOMETIMES / NO

5. **Do you suffer from headaches and/or migraines?**

YES / SOMETIMES / NO

6. **Blood pressure symptoms. Do you have ...**

❋ low blood pressure

❋ high blood pressure

❋ heart palpitations

❋ and/or a quickened pulse after consuming a particular food

YES / SOMETIMES / NO

7. **Musculoskeletal symptoms. Do you have ...**

❋ muscle aches/pains

❋ joint pain

❋ and/or muscle weakness

YES / SOMETIMES / NO

8. **Behavioural changes. Do you have ...**

❋ anxiety

❋ hyperactivity (ADD/ADHD)

❋ temporary confusion

❋ intense cravings (often for the food you are allergic to)

❋ mood changes after eating

❋ and/or sleep problems (excessive need for sleep or insomnia)

YES / SOMETIMES / NO

If you experience three or more allergy symptoms you could have undiagnosed allergies or food/chemical/environmental sensitivities. Other health factors may also be involved so if you have any concerns speak to your doctor for a formal diagnosis. In the meantime, keep a diet diary to help you identify what you ate preceding an attack (for a sample diet diary refer to 'Diet diary', p. 264).

If you have an allergy are you stuck with it for life?

Over the past twenty years, researchers have found that of the 40 per cent of infants and young children with moderate to severe eczema and food allergy, most of their food allergies resolve in early childhood.[18] There is, however, an increased risk of 'atopic march', also known as the 'allergic march'. The atopic march is associated with eczema in early childhood, where the form of allergic response changes over the years. For example, when children under the age of three with eczema and allergies grow out of their allergies, then the more serious symptoms of asthma — wheezing and difficulty of breathing — develop. In the adolescent years, when asthma begins to subside, hay fever symptoms occur. Later in life at about the age of 40, just as allergic rhinitis is settling down, asthma and eczema return.[19] Research shows that antihistamine drugs, which are often prescribed to eczema sufferers, fail to prevent the atopic march.[20] The next section details how diet can alleviate allergy/histamine symptoms and reduce the risk of atopic march.

Recommendations

Eczema sufferers with allergies, especially those with life-threatening anaphylactic reactions, should continue to avoid the offending foods until given clearance by your doctor.

Histamine toxicity

Your body not only makes histamine in response to an allergic reaction, your food also supplies histamines and other amines. According to several research papers, eczema sufferers have elevated histamine levels in the blood combined with a reduced capacity to detoxify these histamines.[21,22,23] And 36 per cent of eczema sufferers experience a worsening of eczema symptoms when they eat amine-rich foods.[24]

Symptoms of histamine toxicity are the same as an allergic reaction: a runny nose or nasal obstruction can be the first signs. Other symptoms include skin rash, a worsening of eczema symptoms, headaches, diarrhoea, stomachache, colic, flatulence, sneezing, asthma and facial flushing.[25] Histamine toxicity occurs when the blood histamine level elevates *beyond what the liver is capable of detoxifying*. Therefore, the health of your liver is an important part of managing allergic reactions and eczema.

The next body of research gives us clues as to how to manage and prevent allergic reactions and reduce the risk of atopic march. In the body, diamine oxidase (DAO) is the main enzyme that breaks down histamine. Monoaminoxidase (MAO) also plays a role in histamine breakdown. According to German researchers, MAO and DAO activity are significantly decreased in patients with atopic eczema, compared with people without eczema.[26] According to research published in the *American Journal of Clinical Nutrition*, DAO activity can be blocked by the consumption of alcohol, food additives, nicotine and heavy metals such as mercury. MAO activity can be blocked by drugs, including some types of antidepressants.[27] Now this is where the research gets interesting: antihistamine medications, which are often prescribed to eczema sufferers, do not improve DAO activity (and antihistamine drugs suppress the liver's ability to detoxify histamines). So while antihistamine drugs mask the symptoms when an allergic reaction occurs, they fail to treat the cause.

While antihistamine drugs can be useful in emergencies, there is a healthy alternative to the daily use of antihistamine drugs, and it comes packaged in the form of papaya. According to research published in the *American Journal of Clinical Nutrition*, vitamin C and vitamin B6 *increase* DAO activity and break down histamine.[28] Laboratory experiments show the flavonoid which is present in onions and available as a supplement, also breaks down histamine.[29,30] (Refer to Table 4, 'Nutrients for liver detoxification', p. 49 and Chapter 6, 'Eczema supplements'.)

Recommendations

- Take natural antihistamines — vitamin C (buffered 'ascorbate' form such as magnesium ascorbate) and vitamin B6 — on a daily basis to reduce the risk of histamine toxicity and allergic reactions.
- Eat papaya, pawpaw (p. 65) and red cabbage (p. 70), as they are rich in vitamin C.

Gastrointestinal tract dysfunction

Like your skin barrier, your gastrointestinal tract is your 'gut barrier' — a vital part of your body's defence system against food-borne bacteria, toxins and allergenic substances.[31] According to Italian researchers, children with eczema often have abnormalities in the gastrointestinal tract, including increased intestinal permeability. A clinical trial revealed 44 per cent of children with atopic eczema have gastrointestinal symptoms after ingesting food (compared with 22 per cent of children without eczema).[32] The most common gastrointestinal symptoms in children with eczema are diarrhoea, regurgitation and vomiting. It's interesting to note that gastrointestinal symptoms were, in most cases, reported to have been present before the appearance of eczema.[33] This research suggests that poor gastrointestinal health can contribute to the appearance of eczema.

According to research published in the *Journal of Investigative Dermatology* and *The Lancet*, eczema sufferers can have increased intestinal permeability, which allows larger food particles, pathogens and toxic substances to enter the body.[34,35] When microbes and toxins pass into your bloodstream, they can block or interfere with biochemical pathways and cause genetic mutations and allergic reactions.

Like a vicious circle, intestinal permeability can also occur *after* you've had an allergic response to food. When a food allergy triggers histamine to be released from mast cells, inflammation and increased vascular permeability occurs. Research shows that the intestinal mucosal defect in eczema sufferers can also exist in eczema patients who don't have food allergies.[36] The following table lists the factors that can cause gastrointestinal damage.

Table 2: Causes of intestinal permeability

alcohol consumption (also damages stomach lining)[37]	consumption of milk and other dairy products (can cause gastrointestinal bleeding in infants)
allergic reactions (histamine release)	frequent chilli consumption (stomach lining damage)
toxic bile	fungal infestation e.g. candidiasis, or parasite infestation
consumption of wheat	consumption of artificial additives (such as preservatives)
excess consumption of salicylates	taking aspirin or non-steroidal anti-inflammatory drugs (NSAIDs)[38]

As you can see, your diet plays a major role in your gastrointestinal health. What happens when you ignore your diet and fail to protect the gut lining from damage? Intestinal permeability creates a heavy workload for the liver, which can lead to damaged liver cells (hepatocytes) and increased free radicals in the bile. In experimental studies, the antioxidant quercetin protects the stomach lining from alcohol-induced damage, if taken during or prior to exposure.[39] The liver is designed to detoxify substances, such as alcohol, and it makes bile to transport toxins to the colon for removal via the faeces. Your diet directly affects how adequately your body eliminates toxin-loaded bile from the colon. The liver produces up to 1 litre of bile salts every day and to do this it needs lecithin from your diet. Your body also needs plenty of dietary fibre to push chemical-loaded bile through the colon and to cleanse the colon of toxic substances, microbes and carcinogens (substances that can cause cancer).

Candida albicans infestation

Another gastrointestinal problem common in eczema sufferers is fungal infestation. Research shows that 70 per cent of patients with atopic eczema have *Candida albicans* overgrowth in the gastrointestinal tract.[40] Furthermore, 69 per cent of infants with seborrhoeic eczema, which affects the scalp, are infected with *Candida albicans* overgrowth at one or more external areas of the skin (including the inside of the mouth).[41] Researchers suggest this may be linked to the use of topical steroid creams (which is another reason why cortisone creams should only be used short-term, if at all). Overgrowth of pathogenic fungus, particularly *Malassezia* and *Candida albicans,* can trigger skin inflammation and increase the incidence of atopic eczema.[42]

What exactly is *Candida albicans*? *Candida albicans* is usually present in the digestive tract and it's a harmless yeast while the immune system keeps it under control. If it proliferates, *Candida albicans* can cause a visible skin infection and it can affect your gastrointestinal tract (infestation can be referred to as candidiasis, yeast infection or thrush). *Candida albicans* overgrowth triggers the production of IgE antibodies (remember how IgE is implicated in allergic reactions? See p. 16). According to research published in *Clinical & Experimental Allergy*, people with atopic eczema and candidiasis are exposed to continuous IgE antibodies, which worsens their eczema symptoms.[43] Unbalanced gut microflora and the proliferation of fungus often come *before* the development of eczema so it is important to treat candida infestation immediately.[44]

Questionnaire 2: *Candida albicans*

Circle any symptom/s you experience on a regular basis, then circle the corresponding answer (YES / SOMETIMES / NO) that best describes the frequency of that symptom or collection of symptoms. YES = weekly or daily; SOMETIMES = monthly or occasionally; NO = never or rarely.

1. **Visible signs of fungal infection on the skin. Do you have ...**
    * red, itchy skin
    * tiny yellow pustules
    * white patches on the skin that show improvement with anti-fungal treatment

    YES / SOMETIMES / NO

2. **Oral signs of candidiasis/yeast infection. Do you have white furry patches inside the mouth?**

    YES / SOMETIMES / NO

3. **Did you have oral thrush as a baby or did your mother have a vaginal thrush infection during pregnancy or birth?**

    YES / NO / UNSURE

4. **Signs of thrush. Do you have ...**
    * genital itching/burning
    * white or chalky discharge or appearance
    * stinging while urinating

    YES / SOMETIMES / NO

5. **Do you take the contraceptive pill or hormone replacement therapy?**

    YES / NO

6. **Have you used steroids/cortisone topically or orally for more than a month?**

    YES / SOMETIMES / NO

7. **Have you required several courses of antibiotics in the last year?**

    YES / NO

8. **Do you crave carbohydrates such as sugar, soft drink, juice, fruit, bread or alcohol?**

    YES / SOMETIMES / NO

9. **Do you need caffeine (coffee, tea, cola, chocolate) each day to 'wake up' or feel good?**

    YES / SOMETIMES / NO

10. **Do you experience stomach bloating after eating?**

    YES / SOMETIMES / NO / UNSURE (List the offending foods, if known:)

    _____

    _____

11. **Have you experienced changes in bowel movements, unpleasant gas or have been diagnosed with inflammatory bowel disease?**

    YES / SOMETIMES / NO

12. **Are you sensitive to perfume, perfumed products, household cleaners and/or cigarette smoke?**

    YES / SOMETIMES / NO / UNSURE

13. **Are you sensitive to chemicals?**

    YES / SOMETIMES / NO / UNSURE

14. **Do rainy days or mouldy environments make you feel unwell?**

    YES / SOMETIMES / NO / UNSURE

15. **Do you have signs of allergies (refer to Questionnaire 1, p. 17)?**

    YES / SOMETIMES / NO / UNSURE

16. **Do you have mood swings (cranky, irritable, aggressive, depressed, angry)?**

    YES / SOMETIMES / NO / UNSURE

17. **Are you hyperactive?**

    YES / SOMETIMES / NO / UNSURE

If you answered yes to any of the physical symptoms (questions 1 to 4) or if you have four or more YES or SOMETIMES answers to questions 5 to 17 then you could have a fungal overgrowth requiring medical treatment. When you have candida overgrowth, eczema symptoms cannot improve, even with a healthy diet, so it is essential to treat the fungal problem. Speak to a pharmacist or doctor about taking a powdered oral anti-fungal and a topical anti-fungal (one that is suitable for eczema). If you are sexually active, your partner should also take an oral anti-fungal (if he has signs of jock itch or if she has signs of thrush, he/she needs to apply a topical anti-fungal for fourteen days and avoid sex during this time). If you have repeatedly suffered from thrush, speak to your doctor about stronger anti-fungal treatments. After you have treated your fungal infection, the Eczema Diet is designed to minimise the risk of further infestations and if you have regular bouts of candidiasis you'll also need to avoid sweet foods like muffins during the Eczema Diet, as fungus proliferates when sugar is in the diet. Also avoid common triggers such as alcohol and tea.

Anti-fungal foods

There are a range of foods that kill fungus in the gastrointestinal tract and these foods include garlic and the onion family, such as eczema-safe leeks and spring onions (scallions).

Do you have worms?

Signs of worm infestation include:

- grinding your teeth at night
- itchy bottom, nose or ears
- children who regularly wet the bed
- frequent nose bleeds
- disturbed sleep (and/or itchy bottom at night)

If you or your child are experiencing signs of worm infestation then speak to your doctor or a pharmacist about oral worming treatments — they are simple, painless and pleasant tasting.

Tip: Remember to always wash your hands before eating to reduce the risk of worms.

Recommendations

- Take a suitable probiotic supplement (for probiotic information see p. 113).
- Ensure you are consuming dietary fibre from pears, rolled oats (porridge, Omega Muesli, p. 214), rice, linseeds, buckwheat and root vegetables, and eat two to three serves of eczema-safe grains daily (see p. 79).
- Drink five to eight glasses of filtered water daily.
- Add garlic, spring onions (scallions), leeks, pawpaw and papaya to your diet.
- Take digestive enzymes, if required.
- Chew your food properly.
- Avoid sugar.
- Avoid milk and other dairy products.
- Avoid drinking alcohol while you have eczema; if you have a rare special occasion when you'd like to have a drink, choose eczema-safe varieties (listed on p. 183) and limit intake to two glasses per fortnight.
- Avoid wheat products for three months.
- If you have signs of intestinal permeability, the amino acid glutamine can help to heal the gut lining, along with probiotics (p. 113), B-group vitamins, vitamin E (p. 108) and magnesium (p. 100). Keep in mind that supplement therapy can fail if you continue to consume gut irritants.

Abnormal fat metabolism

The fats you consume can affect your eczema, so it's important to know a bit about the different types of fats in your diet. Essential fatty acids (EFAs) are polyunsaturated fats and include linoleic acid (commonly known as omega-6) and linolenic acid (which we call omega-3). In general, Western diets are far too low in omega-3 and very high in omega-6, thanks to high intakes of margarine and vegetable oils. It's been estimated that the present Western diet has a ratio of omega-6 to omega-3 of 15:1 (instead of 1:1) and this increases the risk of inflammation.

In the 1930s researchers initially thought that omega-6 was deficient in eczema sufferers. However, research published in the 1980s confirmed the opposite: eczema sufferers tend to have *elevated* omega-6 in their blood and adipose tissue, in conjunction with a decrease in omega-6 metabolites such as DGLA (dihomogamma-linolenic acid).[45] When the milk of nursing mothers was tested, those with *elevated* levels of omega-6 and low levels of DGLA in their milk had children who later went on to develop eczema.[46]

What came first, the eczema or the fat abnormality? A large, carefully designed study by Italian researcher Galli and colleagues demonstrated that the elevated omega-6 and other EFA abnormalities appear before the eczema manifests.[47,48] This suggests that abnormal ratios of essential fatty acids in the diet and/or enzyme blockages caused by diet or stress could be involved in the appearance of eczema.

To promote proper functioning of the enzyme that converts omega-6 (via the FADS2 gene), consume the nutrients biotin, vitamin B6, magnesium and zinc. To promote the conversion of DGLA into skin-smoothing prostaglandins, reduce stress if necessary and avoid consuming trans fats, alcohol and limit high GI foods such as white bread. The mineral chromium helps to reduce high insulin levels after the consumption of carbohydrates.

What are trans fats?

Trans fats are partially or fully hydrogenated fats that act like saturated fats and block some enzyme reactions in the body. For good health, avoid trans fats (check product packaging for phrases like 'trans fats', 'partially hydrogenated oil' or 'hydrogenated oil'). Trans fats are found in cheap vegetable cooking oils, canola oil, doughnuts, pastries, biscuits, Nutella®, chicken nuggets, some margarines, deep fried foods such as fried chicken and hot chips/French fries, imitation cheese, confectionery fats, pizza dough and many fast foods.

What are prostaglandins?

Prostaglandins are hormone-like substances that your body produces to moderate your hormones, your heart, your blood vessels, your cells and they can cause or prevent skin inflammation such as eczema. Prostaglandins are grouped into three families called Series 1, 2 and 3 prostaglandins. Which series a prostaglandin falls into depends on what type of fats you eat — omega-3, omega-6 or saturated fats. See Diagram 3, 'How prostaglandins control inflammation', p. 30.

Recommendations

- To increase omega-3 intake, eat eczema-safe fish once or twice a week (p. 71) and eat linseeds/flaxseeds or use flaxseed oil five times a week (p. 70).
- Reduce saturated fat intake — you can enjoy lean cuts of lamb, veal, turkey and chicken (cut the fat off meats and eat red meat no more than twice a week).
- Avoid trans fats, sausages, deli meats, beef, pork and roast crackling.
- Reduce stress, worry and anxiety, or seek counselling for ways to cope with stress, grief or trauma.
- Greatly reduce omega-6 in the diet (see 'Margarine and vegetable oil', below).
- Don't bother taking an evening primrose oil supplement unless you find it significantly helps your skin (instead, focus on promoting DGLA conversion).
- Take a supplement containing biotin, vitamin B6, zinc and magnesium for delta-6-desaturase enzyme reactions (so the FADS2 gene is more likely to work).
- Take a supplement containing vitamin C and vitamin B3 for delta-5-desaturase enzyme reactions (so the FADS1 gene is more likely to work).
- Eat garlic, leeks and spring onions (scallions). Ginger is allowed in Stage 2 of the diet but not Stage 1.
- Take a supplement containing chromium (see p. 104) and favour low GI foods to reduce insulin production and promote DGLA conversion.

Margarine and vegetable oil

Margarines are made from vegetable oils and have been touted as a healthy alternative to butter, but research is emerging to suggest otherwise. According to a large cross-sectional study in Germany, families who predominantly use margarine (as opposed to butter) are more likely to have children with eczema.[49,50] And frequent consumption of vegetable oils, margarine or frying fats during the last four weeks of pregnancy increases the risk of having a child with eczema.[51] So are these products as healthy as they seem? If you have a look at the ingredient panel of most margarine

Diagram 3: How prostaglandins control inflammation

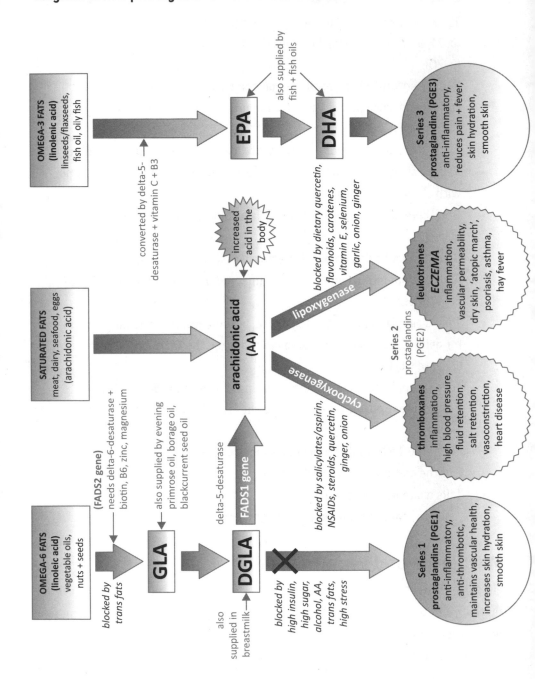

AA (arachidonic acid), DGLA (dihomo-gamma-linolenic acid), EPA (eicos-apentaenoic acid), DHA (docosa-hexaenoic acid), GLA (gamma-linolenic acid), BP (blood pressure), X = blockage of this pathway can contribute to eczema.

tubs and refined vegetable oils, you'll see they contain chemical additives such as preservative 202 and research shows food preservatives cause a worsening of eczema symptoms in more than 50 per cent of eczema sufferers.[52] Margarines usually contain artificial colours, which 40 per cent of you will react to, and antioxidants BHA/320 or 319, which can worsen symptoms in 21 per cent of eczema sufferers.[53] Furthermore, margarines and vegetable oils contain large quantities of omega-6. And despite the marketing hype about the health benefits of margarine and vegetable oils, the fact is the typical western diet is far too rich in omega-6. Our diets are virtually devoid of omega-3 (from seafood, wild/game meats, linseeds/flaxseeds and walnuts) and this disrupts essential fatty acid balance and may partly explain why margarines and vegetable oils increase the risk of eczema.

Recommendations

- Avoid margarine and pastry or baked goods containing margarine.
- Avoid butter in Stage 1 of the Eczema Diet (pure butter is allowed in Stage 2 if you are not allergic to dairy products).
- Limit the amount and types of vegetable oils in the diet (refer to eczema-safe cooking oils on p. 75).

Chemical sensitivity

Chemical sensitivity is an adverse reaction which can occur within 3 hours or up to several days after coming into contact with the offending chemical. How do you know if you have a sensitivity to chemicals? Symptoms are varied and they can be mild to severe depending on the individual and include skin rashes, migraines, headaches, depression, irritability, unfocused behaviour, hyperactivity, flu-like symptoms and a worsening of eczema symptoms. In severe cases, some sensitivities can trigger strong feelings of anger, aggression, suicidal thoughts and physical pain*.

Your diet plays a major role in the appearance of chemical sensitivity, but first let's look at the range of problematic chemicals, which includes natural chemicals such as salicylates, and artificial ones like preservatives, colourings and flavour enhancers.

(*These symptoms can be caused by other factors so speak to your doctor if you are concerned.)

Salicylates

Salicylates are chemicals found in many fruits and vegetables, herbs, nuts, teas, coffee, wine, beer and spices. Salicylates are also in many skin creams and perfumes. According to research by Loblay and Swain from the RPA Hospital Allergy Unit in Sydney, Australia, salicylate sensitivity is the most common chemical sensitivity in eczema sufferers and ingesting salicylate-rich foods can cause a worsening of eczema symptoms.[54] A high dose of salicylates (especially if taking aspirin, which contains salicylates) can cause temporary damage to the stomach lining, especially in children and sensitive individuals.

Salicylates are often touted as an eczema sufferer's worst enemy, but are they to be permanently avoided? Maybe not. Salicylates are often found in the most nutritious foods such as dark leafy green vegetables and blueberries so you want to do all you can to prevent or decrease salicylate sensitivity. Here is the key: your liver is designed to detoxify salicylates and other chemicals so they can be safely removed from the body. In order for this to occur, your diet (or the maternal diet if your eczema-prone baby is being breastfed), needs to supply *all* the nutrients the liver requires for salicylate detoxification. These nutrients are glycine[55], vitamin B6 and magnesium.

Although it is not essential, you can test to see how well your liver is processing salicylates by using a liver function test home kit (where you take aspirin, so if you are allergic to aspirin this test is not suitable for you). See 'Resources', p. 265, for more information. There is more information on salicylates and liver detoxification of chemicals coming up shortly.

Recommendations

- It's essential for eczema sufferers to supplement with the correct doses of glycine, magnesium and vitamin B6 (see Chapter 6, 'Eczema supplements').
- Greatly reduce salicylate intake (some healthy salicylate foods are essential in the diet and these include carrots, sweet potato and fresh beetroot as they supply carotenoids for skin protection).
- Avoid aspirin* and baby teething gels as they are rich in salicylates (for alternatives to teething gel refer to p. 153). (*If you have been

prescribed aspirin for heart disease, do not stop taking aspirin, and talk to your doctor about your options. Do not take glycine if you are on blood thinning medications such as aspirin.)

Nitrates

Nitrates are chemicals used to preserve meats such as bacon, sausages and ham. In the 1970s it was discovered that during the cooking of nitrate-containing meats, harmful nitrosamines form which can cause cancer and liver damage.[56,57,58] It is for this reason government health authorities in Australia recommend we don't eat deli meats or sausages. Carcinogenic nitrosamines are present in tobacco smoke and in the nettings wrapped around deli meats such as ham, which can contaminate the meat.[59,60] According to research by Loblay and Swain, eczema sufferers are sensitive to nitrates and nitrate consumption can worsen eczema symptoms in 43 per cent of eczema sufferers.[61]

Your diet can help to reduce the damaging effects of nitrates. According to laboratory studies, the antioxidants quercetin, vitamin C and vitamin E help to reverse the liver damage caused by nitrate consumption.[62,63,64]

Recommendations

- Avoid nitrate-containing meats as they increase cancer risk and eczema symptoms.
- Ensure your diet contains the antioxidants quercetin, vitamin C and vitamin E (see Chapter 6, 'Eczema supplements').

Food colourings

If you've ever eaten food at a children's party, chances are you have ingested dozens of artificial food colourings known to exacerbate eczema. And it's not just brightly coloured party food, either. Regular breakfast cereal, yoghurt and margarines contain colourings that can trigger a range of adverse reactions, including a worsening of eczema symptoms.[65]

Tartrazine (102), one of several yellow food colourings, worsens eczema symptoms in 40 per cent of eczema sufferers and it can trigger asthma attacks, a runny nose, purplish skin bruising and in severe cases anaphylactic shock. How can eating a yellow lolly cause such problems? Tartrazine stimulates the production of pro-inflammatory leukotrienes. A team of researchers at Southampton University in the United Kingdom also found that artificial colourings could hamper a child's intelligence by up to five IQ points and cause behavioural problems such as inattention and hyperactivity.[66]

Artificial colourings are not the only additives eczema sufferers should avoid. There is a natural food colouring that is problematic for eczema-prone people and most children are consuming it on a daily basis. Annatto (160b), used to colour many brands of butter, yoghurt and fish fingers to name a few, can cause eczema flare-ups in sensitive individuals. Adverse reactions to annatto include obsessive head banging, irritable bowel syndrome, headaches, learning difficulties and (surprisingly) some children may obsessively favour yellow: for example, they only want yellow food/pencils/clothes, which ceases when annatto is removed from the diet.[67] In Europe, annatto has been banned from use in foods and a safe alternative, beta-carotene (160a), is used. A range of problematic colourants are listed in 'Additives to avoid', below.

Table 3: Additives to avoid

Additive	Number/s	Food sources
flavour enhancers: glutamates, monosodium glutamate (MSG)	620–635	flavoured noodles, chicken-salted chips, flavoured crackers and crisps, sauces, stock cubes, gravies, fast foods, traditional Chinese cooking (natural sources of MSG include tomato, soy sauce, broccoli, mushrooms, spinach, grapes, plums, deli meats, miso, tempeh, wine, rum, sherry, brandy, liqueur)
artificial colourings: tartrazine (yellow), red, blue, green, black, brown	102, 104, 107, 110, 122–129, 132, 133, 142, 151, 155 (US: blue 1 and 2, green 3, red 2, 3, 4 and 40, yellow 5 and 6)	confectionery/lollies/candy, jelly, breakfast cereals, glacé cherries, salmon, hot dogs, soft drinks, flavoured mineral water, chocolate, potato crisps, corn chips, toppings, ice-cream, iceblocks (popsicles/ice lollies), fruit drinks, cordials, flavoured milks, meat pies, cupcakes, cakes, liqueur, yoghurt and dairy snacks
natural colouring	160b (annatto)	in many yoghurts, butter, fish fingers, custard and commercial desserts (160a is a safe alternative)

Additive	Number/s	Food sources
preservatives	sorbates 200–203 benzoates 210–213 sulfites 220–228 nitrates, nitrites 249–252 propionates 280–283	used in some processed fruits and vegetables, wines, beer, most soft drinks (sodas), diet drinks, cordials, juices, processed meats, sausages, dried fruit, processed deli meats (e.g. sausages, devon, ham, salami); 282 in some breads, buns and wraps
antioxidant preservatives	310–321	in oils, margarines, chips, fried snack foods, fast foods
artificial sweeteners: aspartame, saccharin	951, 954	NutraSweet®, Equal®, Sweet 'N Low®, diet and 'sugar-free' products, diet soft drinks (sodas), 'zero' soft drinks, cakes, cookies, sweet pies, muffins, ice-creams

Sources: McCann, D. et al., 2007, 'Food additives and hyperactive behaviour in 3-year-old and 8/9-year-old children in the community: a randomised, double-blinded, placebo-controlled trial', *The Lancet,* vol. 370, pp. 1560–7; Dengate, S., Food Intolerance Network fact sheet, retrieved 12 May 2011: www.fedup.com.au

Recommendations

- Avoid artificial chemicals, especially food colourings, preservatives and flavour enhancers.
- Avoid natural colour annatto (160b).
- Refer to the handy shopping guides in Part 3 for a list of additives to avoid when you are grocery shopping ('Eczema-safe shopping guide: Stage 1' is on pp. 260–261).

Brewer's yeast

Approximately 31 per cent of eczema sufferers have a worsening of eczema symptoms after consuming brewer's yeast.[68] Brewer's yeast is a fungal micro-organism used to ferment carbohydrates in beer and it is available as a nutrition supplement.

Sulfites

Sulfites, such as sulphur dioxide, are food preservatives which are commonly used to preserve wines, deli meats, dried fruits and dried vegetables, to name a few. Sulfites destroy vitamin B1 and folic acid in foods so they can be considered an 'anti-nutrient' (anti-nutrients are discussed on p. 60). While dried fruits might be touted as a healthy snack for children, one dried apricot can contain 16mg of sulphur dioxide which can cause a worsening of eczema symptoms in susceptible individuals and/or a range of adverse reactions such as diarrhoea, unfocused behaviour, hyperactivity, smelly gas and it could trigger an asthma attack in susceptible individuals.[69]

If you've ever experienced facial flushing after drinking a glass of red wine or consuming vinegar you may be sensitive to sulfites, and highly sensitive people may react to sulphur-rich garlic and onions.

Monosodium glutamate (MSG)

A study conducted by Loblay and Swain found that 35 per cent of eczema sufferers have adverse reactions to monosodium glutamate, a flavour enhancer that is both natural (present in tomato) and artificial (in products such as flavoured potato chips). Dietary MSG can not only worsen eczema symptoms, it may increase the risk of premature wrinkles because it reduces stores of glutathione, an anti-ageing antioxidant enzyme needed for liver detoxification of chemicals.[70] In animal studies, MSG ingestion promotes liver inflammation, which significantly increases the size of the liver and promotes liver damage.[71]

Can modifying your diet make up for previous dietary sins? Clinical studies show MSG-induced liver damage can be reversed with antioxidant supplementation.[72]

Reduce your chemical load

Consuming soy sauce, fermented soybeans, chocolate, cheese, coffee and yoghurt causes a worsening of eczema symptoms, according to a Japanese study published in the *Journal of Dermatology*. After the avoidance of these foods for three months all the participating eczema sufferers had reduced eczema symptoms.[73]

Recommendations

- Avoid consuming artificial additives in your diet.
- Wash fruits and vegetables in water, soaking them for several minutes. Use a soft scrubbing brush on hardy fruits and vegetables and peel the skin where possible.
- For more information on avoiding chemicals, read Chapter 8, 'General recommendations for eczema'.
- Additives to avoid are listed in the handy shopping guides, on pp. 260–263.
- While you have eczema, avoid natural MSG sources such as soy sauce, tomato and grapes (for a list of foods containing MSG refer to Table 3, 'Additives to avoid', p. 34).
- Avoid artificial MSG and other flavour enhancers.
- Avoid sulfite-rich foods and drinks, including dried fruits and alcohol (sulfite-rich foods are listed in Table 3, 'Additives to avoid' p. 34).
- Supplement with the antioxidants vitamin C, vitamin E and alpha-lipoic acid (supplement details are in Chapter 6).

Lactose + dairy products

Lactose is the sugar portion of dairy products such as cow's milk, yoghurt, butter and cheese. In order for your body to break down lactose, you require the enzyme lactase in your digestive tract. If you are sensitive to dairy products it is likely that your body does not adequately produce this enzyme. Lactose intolerance can cause diarrhoea, gas, cramps and bloating. More than 40 per cent of eczema sufferers are sensitive to lactose and they experience a worsening of eczema symptoms when they consume lactose.[74]

It's not only lactose intolerance that can occur. A total of 38 per cent of eczema sufferers are allergic to cow's milk and dairy products.[75] Aside from diagnosed allergies, dairy products can cause damage to the lining of the gastrointestinal tract. Research shows the consumption of cow's milk causes gastrointestinal bleeding in 50 per cent of American infants who present with iron deficiency (frequent milk consumption can also cause iron-deficiency anaemia). When the gut lining is damaged from eating dairy products, tiny holes allow larger food particles to enter the body and allergic reactions can result. Naturopaths often refer to this as 'leaky gut syndrome' and the medical term is 'increased intestinal permeability'. A dairy-free diet is one of the most effective ways to decrease the appearance of eczema, even when dairy allergy or lactose intolerance is not present.

Recommendations

- Avoid all dairy products while you have eczema and refer to the calcium information on p. 117.

Questionnaire 3: Eczema + diet

The following questionnaire is suitable for adults and children with eczema, and if you have a baby with eczema you can use this questionnaire to assess maternal diet (the diet of the mother during pregnancy and/or the diet of both parents before conception).

Circle the foods you consume and then circle the corresponding answer (YES / SOMETIMES / NO) that best describes the frequency of consumption. YES = weekly or daily; SOMETIMES = monthly or occasionally; NO = never.

Part 1. Do you ...

1. eat raw egg or raw egg whites?
   YES / SOMETIMES / NO

2. have whole-egg mayonnaise in your fridge?
   YES / SOMETIMES / NO

3. eat mayonnaise, coleslaw or creamy salad dressings?
   YES / SOMETIMES / NO

4. drink protein shakes containing powdered/fresh egg or egg whites?
   YES / SOMETIMES / NO

5. eat hollandaise sauce or eggs Benedict?
   YES / SOMETIMES / NO

6. eat the icing on traditional wedding cakes?
   YES / SOMETIMES / NO

7. have mood disturbances such as depression, moodiness or anxiety?
   YES / SOMETIMES / NO

8. eat traditional chocolate mousse? (store-bought varieties may not contain egg but they have lots of artificial additives)
   YES / SOMETIMES / NO

9. have dermatitis plus any of the following symptoms: greyish pallor of the skin, scaly lips, nausea, loss of appetite, muscle pain, raised cholesterol or localised numbness?
   YES / SOMETIMES / NO

10. eat store-bought dips containing egg (e.g. baba ganoush/tuna/beetroot)? (not including hummus, tahini or pesto-type dips)
    YES / SOMETIMES / NO

Part 2. Do you ...

11. use margarine?
    YES / SOMETIMES / NO

12. consume store-bought pastry or softened butter (containing vegetable oil and additives)?
    YES / SOMETIMES / NO

13. use canola oil, plain vegetable oil, olive oil or 'light' cooking oil?
    YES / SOMETIMES / NO

14. eat fried foods (e.g. takeaway/takeout foods cooked in oil, or fish and chips)?
    YES / SOMETIMES / NO

Part 3. Do you ...

15. eat a lot of fruit? (3 pieces/1½ cups or more per day)
    YES / SOMETIMES / NO

16. frequently eat broad beans, broccoli, cauliflower, eggplant (aubergine), gherkins, olives, mushrooms, silver beet or spinach?
    YES / SOMETIMES / NO

17. frequently eat tomato, oranges, lemon, kiwi fruit or strawberries?
    YES / SOMETIMES / NO

18. drink tea, herbal tea or coffee?
    YES / SOMETIMES / NO

19. drink tomato juice, flavoured soft drink/sodas or cordial?
    YES / SOMETIMES / NO

20. drink beer, wine, cider, brandy, liqueur, port, rum or sherry?
    YES / SOMETIMES / NO

21. eat cornflakes or consume corn products?
    YES / SOMETIMES / NO

22. have adverse reactions to aspirin?
    YES / SOMETIMES / NO

23. use teething gel (babies and toddlers)
    YES / SOMETIMES / NO

Part 4. Do you …

24. eat grapes, plums, prunes, raisins, sultanas, tomato and/or tomato products such as sauces and juice?

    YES / SOMETIMES / NO

25. eat broccoli, mushrooms, silver beet or spinach?

    YES / SOMETIMES / NO

26. eat deli meats such as devon, turkey, chicken, salami and sausages?

    YES / SOMETIMES / NO

27. consume gravy, soy sauce, flavoured potato chips/crisps or flavoured rice crackers?

    YES / SOMETIMES / NO

28. drink wine, brandy, liqueur, port, rum or sherry?

    YES / SOMETIMES / NO

Part 5. Do you …

29. chew gum or use mouth wash?

    YES / SOMETIMES / NO

30. consume flavoured potato chips/crisps, diet soft drink/soda, cordial, flavoured rice crackers, coloured iceblocks/popsicles/ice lollies, flavoured corn chips or sweets?

    YES / SOMETIMES / NO

Analysis of Questionnaire 3

Let's take a look at the results of Questionnaire 3 to identify where you might need to alter your diet.

Part 1: egg white injury

Assess your total intake of raw egg whites. If you consume whole-egg mayonnaise once a week, tuna dip once a week and hollandaise sauce once a week, this is classified as frequent consumption of raw egg white and egg white injury may result. Egg white injury and biotin information is on p. 96.

Part 2: vegetable oil

If you consume margarine, products containing margarine, or vegetable oils, discontinue use and refer to the rice bran oil information on p. 75.

Part 3: salicylates

This section highlights foods and drinks rich in salicylates. Do not consume these products while on the Eczema Diet as doing so may affect your results (if you have been prescribed aspirin for heart disease do not stop taking aspirin, and talk to your doctor about your options).

Part 4: MSG and flavour enhancers

This section highlights foods and drinks rich in natural MSG and foods containing artificial flavour enhancers. Do not consume these products while on the Eczema Diet as doing so may affect your results.

Part 5: artificial chemicals (general)

Do not consume these products while on the Eczema Diet.

Chapter 3

Healthy liver, healthy skin

The liver is the second largest organ in the body (after the skin) and it performs a range of important body functions which can greatly affect the appearance of your skin. Your liver filters more than 1½ litres (approximately 3 pints) of blood per minute and receives a dual blood supply: one containing freshly oxygenated blood from the heart, and the other supplying blood from the stomach and intestines, rich with newly absorbed nutrients from your diet, as well as toxins, microbes, drugs and hormones. The liver plays a vital role in detoxifying these substances so the blood remains healthy and it assists with supplying the body with nutrients for beautiful skin.

Fatty liver, where your liver accumulates fat and enlarges, can occur in eczema patients. According to research by Dr Kimata from the Department of Pediatrics and Allergy at the Ujitakeda Hospital in Kyoto (Japan), more than 17 per cent of non-obese children with eczema also have fatty liver. This result is significantly high compared to 3.2 per cent of *non-atopic* children, 3.7 per cent of *hay fever* sufferers and 5 per cent of asthma sufferers who have fatty liver. Dr Kimata's research showed that atopic eczema is also associated with fat malabsorption, nutritional deficiencies and eating trans fats, all of which can affect liver health.

Detoxification, a brief history

When a medical drug is prescribed to a patient, what happens to that drug once it enters the body? Over the centuries, the study of detoxification has been undertaken by scientists to help answer this question. It was back in the 1700s that scientists first hypothesised that after a toxin was consumed it was transformed into a water-soluble substance and removed from the body via the urine. And in 1842, in a detoxification experiment, Keller proved this theory, using an amino acid supplement called glycine. In 1947, in *Detoxification Mechanisms*, R.T. Williams defined for the first time the two separate phases of detoxification. Today the scientific research on liver detoxification of toxins is an essential part of drug safety testing done by pharmaceutical companies to reduce the risk of people overdosing while taking prescription drugs. This research on liver detoxification can also help you to be eczema-free.

Phase 1 liver detoxification (and why it can make your skin worse)

Food and chemical sensitivities can indicate that your Phase 1 and/or Phase 2 detoxification pathways are imbalanced. Most drugs and food chemicals are processed through a Phase 1 reaction involving cytochrome P450 enzymes. Their role is to make toxic substances water-soluble so they can be further processed during Phase 2 of liver detoxification. Williams found that in some cases during Phase 1 liver detoxification, chemicals could become more toxic than the original substances (he thought the term detoxification could be misleading in these instances). The findings were of great importance because before this time therapeutic agents (such as pharmaceutical drugs) were being prescribed without doctors being aware of the metabolic fate of the drug once a patient had swallowed it.[1] Malfunctioning Phase 1 or Phase 2 liver detoxification reactions have been implicated in adverse reactions to drugs.[2]

Phase 1 can greatly increase free radical production, which can damage DNA and cause genetic mutations *if your diet is not rich in antioxidants*. When Phase 1 detoxification is high you can experience a worsening of symptoms and you may feel lethargic, and it is around this time that antihistamine drugs are often prescribed. Antihistamine medications can make you temporarily feel better as they can mask the symptoms, but there is a catch: antihistamine medications *temporarily* block Phase 1 liver detoxification. This is not ideal as blocking liver detoxification reactions creates an increased workload for your kidneys *and* your skin as both are left with the task of chemical waste elimination.

While antihistamine drugs can be useful in emergencies, there are natural alternatives to antihistamine drugs which can be used on a daily basis. As mentioned in Chapter 2, vitamin C, vitamin B6 and quercetin are natural antihistamines that can prevent histamine toxicity. You can also help to minimise the potentially damaging effects of Phase 1 by consuming a diet rich in antioxidants vitamin C, vitamin E, quercetin and alpha-lipoic acid.

Phase 1 blockers

Phase 1 detoxification is reduced by antihistamine drugs, benzodiazepines (anti-anxiety drugs), ketoconazole (an anti-fungal drug), fluconazole (Diflucan®, an anti-fungal drug), erythromycin (an antibiotic), acid blockers (anti-ulcer medications), grapefruit (it contains a compound called naringenin which reduces cytochrome P450 activity) and the liver-protective herb St Mary's Thistle. While short-term blockage of Phase 1 can be useful to temporarily relieve symptoms, long-term use of these substances can be problematic as reduced liver detoxification function can burden the kidneys.

Phase 2 liver detoxification (and why it can prevent chemical sensitivity)

Instead of blocking Phase 1 detoxification, there is a much healthier solution: boost Phase 2 detoxification. In Phase 2, a toxin that has been partly processed in Phase 1, joins with a substance, such as an amino acid, so it can be safely removed via the urine or bile. For example, eczema sufferers are often sensitive to salicylates which can worsen eczema symptoms. During Phase 2 detoxification, between 55 and 60 per cent of dietary salicylates are joined with the amino acid glycine, allowing salicylates to be removed from the body (this is one of the reasons why glycine is effective at reducing eczema symptoms). Without this glycine-joining step, salicylates can re-enter the bloodstream and accumulate, leading to salicylate sensitivity. Preservatives, toxic heavy metals, histamines, amines and other chemicals, both natural and artificial, are also processed during Phase 2 liver detoxification.

The following questionnaire highlights other symptoms that can indicate your liver detoxification function needs dietary support. This questionnaire is suitable for adults and children. If you have a baby with eczema, you can use this questionnaire to assess maternal diet (the diet of the mother during pregnancy and/or the diet of both parents before conception).

Recommendations

- Your diet can help to reverse or prevent fatty liver: limit or avoid drinking alcohol, maintain a healthy weight, reduce fat intake and add lecithin to your diet. Lecithin contains choline, which breaks down fats so they don't accumulate in the liver (read 'Lecithin granules', p. 74).

- Avoid trans fats and prevent or reverse nutritional deficiencies with supplementation.
- Take liver detoxification nutrients to promote healthy liver function.

Questionnaire 4: Liver detoxification

Circle any symptom/s you experience on a regular basis and then circle the corresponding answer (YES / SOMETIMES / NO) that best describes the frequency of that symptom or collection of symptoms. YES = weekly or daily; SOMETIMES = monthly or occasionally; NO = never or rarely.

Do you have …

1. **dry and/or itchy skin?**
   YES / SOMETIMES / NO

2. **intolerance to greasy foods (e.g. diarrhoea after taking omega-3 tablets or feeling unwell/diarrhoea after a greasy meal)?**
   YES / SOMETIMES / NO

3. **foul smelling stools?**
   YES / SOMETIMES / NO

4. **headaches after eating?**
   YES / SOMETIMES / NO

5. **hypoglycaemia or low blood sugar or fatigue/energy crashes or sleepiness after eating?**
   YES / SOMETIMES / NO

6. **cravings for stimulants (e.g. coffee, chocolate, sweets)?**
   YES / SOMETIMES / NO

7. **constipation?**
   YES / SOMETIMES / NO

8. pallor/greyish/dull looking skin?

   YES / SOMETIMES / NO

9. yellow in whites of eyes?

   YES / SOMETIMES / NO

10. bad breath or unpleasant body odour?

    YES / SOMETIMES / NO

11. pain in right side under ribcage?

    YES / SOMETIMES / NO

12. water retention/oedema?

    YES / SOMETIMES / NO

13. sour taste in your mouth?

    YES / SOMETIMES / NO

14. high blood cholesterol: cholesterol over 200 mg/dl or 5.5 (CDN)?

    YES / UNKNOWN / NO

15. previously had jaundice?

    YES / UNKNOWN / NO

16. hepatitis?

    YES / UNKNOWN / NO

17. nausea?

    YES / SOMETIMES / NO

18. depression/moodiness/fluctuating moods?

    YES / SOMETIMES / NO

19. allergies/hives/hay fever/high blood histamine level or allergic shiners
    (dark circles under eyes)?

    YES / SOMETIMES / NO

20. **gallstones?**
    YES / SOMETIMES / NO

21. **chronic fatigue syndrome?**
    YES / SOMETIMES / NO

22. **intolerance to alcohol, antibiotics or drugs?**
    YES / SOMETIMES / NO

23. **intolerance to aspirin or salicylates or baby teething gel?**
    YES / UNKNOWN / NO

24. **chemical/food sensitivities?**
    YES / UNKNOWN / NO

25. **sulfite sensitivity or sensitivity to wine, dried fruit and vinegar?**
    YES / UNKNOWN / NO

Analysis of Questionnaire 4

If you have fewer than two symptoms, then taking supplements would be optional (but highly recommended) while on the Eczema Diet. If you answered yes to three or more questions, you should take supplements while on the Eczema Diet. There is a test that measures how well your Phase 1 and Phase 2 liver detoxification reactions are working (listed in 'Resources', p. 265). On saying this, if you have eczema, it is a sign that Phase 1 and Phase 2 are imbalanced and nutritional support is required.

Your liver is the body's main chemical processing organ to remove chemicals, histamines and toxins. *No drug can ever replace the nutrients required for liver detoxification of these substances.* A healthy diet and antioxidants support liver function. What are the specific nutrients needed for liver detoxification of chemicals? Here is the list.

Table 4: Nutrients for liver detoxification

Sensitivities/ adverse reactions to:	Phase 2 liver detoxification pathway	Nutrients and foods required
amines (e.g. from meat, frozen fish, deli meats, nitrosamines) fungal toxins, pickled foods, high oestrogen	glucuronidation (metabolises 33% of drugs such as paracetamol and NSAIDs, and deactivates sex hormones especially oestrogens, food oestrogens)	magnesium, zinc, B group vitamins, ground turmeric (spice), essential fatty acids (omega-3) (+ reduce dietary amines)
histamines, histamine toxicity (also see sulfation pathway)	other mechanisms	vitamin C, vitamin B6, quercetin, taurine, methionine, cysteine (possibly magnesium and CoEnzyme Q10)
pesticide exposure, toxic heavy metals, penicillin, alcohol, paracetamol	glutathionation (anti-ageing if it works well)	brussels sprouts, cabbage (and other cruciferous veg.), glycine, glutamine, cysteine, methionine, vitamin B2, vitamin B6, vitamin C, selenium, glutathione (+ avoid toxic heavy metals)
salicylates (salicylic acids, aspirin, teething gel) MSG (tomato, Chinese takeaway, flavour enhanced savoury foods e.g. chips/crisps) sulfites (additives in wine, vinegar) tartrazine (yellow food colouring, 102) preservatives (210–213)	glycination	glycine, magnesium, vitamin B6, taurine (+ reduce dietary salicylates)
food histamines, sulfites	sulfation	molybdenum (co-factor for sulphur oxidase), vitamin B12, vitamin B6, folic acid/folate, sulphur-containing foods e.g. garlic, onion and cabbage (avoid additives 220–228, preserved meats, deli meats, pickled foods, vinegar, dried fruits, alcohol esp. wine)

Recommendations

- Consume the nutrients required for Phase 2 liver detoxification function (refer to Table 4, 'Nutrients for liver detoxification' p. 49).
- Reduce intake of salicylates, amines and histamine-rich foods as they create a heavy workload for your liver, kidneys and skin.
- Refer to Chapter 6, 'Eczema supplements'.

Acid–alkaline balance

There is another way to help your liver detoxify problematic chemicals: by consuming foods that have an alkalising effect in the body. Keeping your diet in acid–alkaline balance promotes healthy blood and strong bones and it gives your skin a healthy glow. Do you remember learning about acids and bases at school? Your food does more than stop the hunger pangs and boost your energy; once your meal is digested it releases either an acid or an alkaline base into your bloodstream. Your blood needs to be slightly alkaline at a pH between 7.35 and 7.45 to be healthy and your body will do all it can to keep the blood within these limits (more on this in a moment). pH means 'potential of hydrogen' and on the pH scale 0 is strongly acidic, 7 is neutral and up to 14 is strongly alkaline.[3]

Alkalisation, a brief history

Alkalisation is the term used for the administration of highly alkalising foods or supplements for a short period of time, such as during a 'detox'. In the seventeenth century the first medical experiments regarding the body's balance of acids and alkalis were conducted.[4] Doctors also used alkalisation to treat a range of health problems, including gout. In the mid 1900s the body's acid–alkaline balance became popular for its role in the detoxification of chemicals.[5] Salicylate sensitivity is the most common chemical sensitivity that eczema sufferers have, and back in the 1950s alkalisation was used as an effective treatment for eliminating salicylates from the body.[6,7] In 1955, according to Gutman in the *Journal of Clinical Investigation*, medical staff at hospitals used alkalisation to treat salicylate poisoning from accidental aspirin overdose*.[8] Alkalisation also supports detoxification of chemicals such as preservatives, amines, food colourings and MSG. (*When the urine pH exceeds an alkaline reading of 7.5, more salicylates are eliminated than reabsorbed, and three times the amount of salicylates are excreted via the urine.)

The Eczema Diet includes a 3-day Alkalising Cleanse, which is a liver detox and gastrointestinal cleansing program designed specifically for adults with eczema and chemical sensitivities. While this is a nutritious alkalisation program for short-term use, for everyday health your daily diet needs to have *acid–alkaline balance*. While some of the recipes in the Eczema Diet are highly alkalising, such as Tarzan Juice (p. 222), Healthy Skin Juice (p. 222) and Alkaline Bomb Salad (p. 233), most of the recipes are classed as acid–alkaline balanced because they contain both alkalising and healthy acid-producing ingredients so they meet your body's nutritional needs for protein, fibre, minerals, essential fatty acids and so on.

The following is a brief list of alkalising, neutral and acidifying foods; for the full list refer to Chapter 19, 'Eczema-safe food charts', p. 252.

Alkalising	Acidifying
vegetables	tap water (non-filtered)
herbs	protein foods, meat, seafood and beans/legumes
all sprouts and sprouted grains	all grains (non-sprouted)
rice malt syrup	corn
apple cider vinegar	peanuts
a few fruits such as banana, lemon and lime	most fruits
pure springwater (not carbonated)	sugar
	all sweeteners (except rice malt syrup)
	artificial additives
Neutral	soft drink (sodas)
filtered water	alcohol
	caffeine products
	most vinegars (except apple cider vinegar)

Acidifying diets

The standard American or Western diet is unbalanced as it largely consists of acid-producing ingredients. Modern diets are generally high in protein and refined grains and low in alkalising vegetables and it's well documented that these diets cause chronic, low-grade metabolic acidosis that worsens with age as kidney function declines.[9,10,11,12] What happens when your daily diet is constantly acid-producing? Let's say you consume a beef burger containing red meat, bacon, tomato sauce and lettuce, and you wash it down with a glass of Diet Coke® or a cup of coffee. Once digested, this meal floods acids into your bloodstream and your body responds by releasing calcium (which is alkaline) into your bloodstream. This usually ensures the blood's pH returns to alkaline and it is an important process that keeps you alive.

Is the problem solved? Not exactly. Your meal has depleted some of your calcium stores, and where does your body get calcium from? Calcium can be taken from the body's reserves and leached from your bones. Excess acids can be excreted via the skin, lungs and kidneys, which can burden these systems. Acids can be stored in your tissues, which can make the skin itchy. Research shows the consumption of Western acidifying diets causes weakened bones, muscle wasting, kidney stone formation and damage to the kidneys.[13,14,15]

How to monitor your pH

Your pH changes throughout the day as each meal and drink influences your blood, urine, saliva and tissue pH readings. You can test your urine and saliva pH at home, several times a day if you wish, using a pH test kit containing litmus paper (these test kits are available from some health food shops and online). The saliva test measures your body tissue pH and it should be done about 30 minutes after eating or drinking. When you test your urine pH (this is the preferred test) the amount of acids your kidneys are excreting is measured. It is useful to monitor your pH several times a day, for at least two weeks, so you can see for yourself how your diet affects your pH (also keep in mind that stress can cause an acid reading). If you note that you are particularly acidic, you can eat or drink one of the double star rated recipes ★ ★ to help restore acid–alkaline balance.

The following questionnaire is suitable for adults and children. If you have a baby with eczema, you can use this questionnaire to assess maternal diet (the diet of the mother during pregnancy and/or the diet of both parents before conception).

Questionnaire 5: Acid–alkaline balance

Circle any foods and beverages you consume on a regular basis (or any symptom) and/or circle the corresponding answer (YES / SOMETIMES / NO).
YES = weekly or daily; SOMETIMES = monthly or occasionally; NO = never.
Do you ...

1. eat fewer than five serves (2½ cups) of vegetables daily?
   YES / SOMETIMES / NO

2. eat processed deli meats and/or smoked meats?
   YES / SOMETIMES / NO

3. eat beef, sausages and/or pork?
   YES / SOMETIMES / NO

4. drink caffeine (coffee, tea, chocolate milk) daily?
   YES / SOMETIMES / NO

5. eat processed breakfast cereal?
   YES / SOMETIMES / NO

6. add sugar to foods or drinks (e.g. with coffee, tea or cereal)?
   YES / SOMETIMES / NO

7. eat pickled vegetables e.g. gherkins?
   YES / SOMETIMES / NO

8. eat cheese and/or sweetened fruit-flavoured yoghurt?
   YES / SOMETIMES / NO

9. eat dried packet soup mixes?

    YES / SOMETIMES / NO

10. eat commercial tomato sauce or barbecue sauce?

    YES / SOMETIMES / NO

11. eat ice-cream and/or custard?

    YES / SOMETIMES / NO

12. regularly eat corn or corn products?

    YES / SOMETIMES / NO

13. eat lots of fruit?

    YES / SOMETIMES / NO

14. take medical drugs or recreational drugs?

    YES / SOMETIMES / NO

15. eat chocolate?

    YES / SOMETIMES / NO

16. eat peanuts or peanut butter?

    YES / SOMETIMES / NO

17. drink alcohol and/or soft drink (sodas)?

    YES / SOMETIMES / NO

18. consume artificial sweetener?

    YES / SOMETIMES / NO

19. eat desserts?

    YES / SOMETIMES / NO

20. eat white flour products (e.g. white bread, baked goods)?

    YES / SOMETIMES / NO

21. **use margarine or softened butter containing additives?**
YES / SOMETIMES / NO

22. **have regular bouts of *Candida albicans* overgrowth/yeast infection?**
YES / SOMETIMES / NO

Analysis of Questionnaire 5

If you answered yes to three or more questions, your diet is likely to be acidifying and contributing to your eczema. However, if you drink a cup of coffee or tea, or a glass of alcohol or soft drink every day your pH reading is likely to be highly acidic.

Please keep in mind that it is not necessary, or recommended, to follow a 100 per cent alkalising diet for more than a week at a time. There are many acid-forming foods, such as legumes and wholegrains, which are important for healthy skin, and if you like eating meat you can enjoy it in moderation (with the fat carefully cut off or drained). On saying this, if you can avoid red meat and favour legumes, skinless chicken and eczema-safe varieties of fish this would be ideal. Your aim is to eat a healthy, balanced diet that contains both alkaline and nutritious acid-forming foods.

Balanced meals

Here are some examples of lunch box items that are acidifying and rich in chemicals that can worsen eczema symptoms:

Lunch box 1: wholemeal sandwich using bread to suit your allergies, strawberries, additive-free muesli (granola) bar and organic fruit yoghurt.
Why is this lunch box a bad choice? This lunch box seems healthy but every item is acid-producing, and nothing is alkalising, and it could cause a flare-up thanks to the natural chemicals present in the fruits.

Lunch box 2: ham sandwich on white bread with margarine, orange, cheese, fruit-flavoured yoghurt, cake or biscuits and chocolate milk.
Why is this lunch box a bad choice? Every item is strongly acid-producing and rich in irritating chemicals, so this lunch box would cause your eczema to flare up (and it could be severe).

Here are some examples of eczema-safe lunch boxes:

Lunch box 3: wholemeal salad sandwich using bread to suit your allergies, with iceberg lettuce, grated carrot and mung bean sprouts, pear muffin (homemade), plain rice crackers and baked banana chips (homemade), celery sticks and filtered water.

Why is this lunch box a good choice? Celery and salad ingredients are alkalising, sprouts are strongly alkalising (bonus points for this item), the other foods are healthy acid-producing items and filtered water is neutral.

Lunch box 4: free-range chicken and lettuce wrap (using spelt lavash bread/flat bread), banana, carrot sticks, brown rice crackers and filtered water.

Why is this lunch box a good choice? Carrot, lettuce and banana are alkalising and the chicken, bread and crackers are acid-forming but they are also eczema-safe and supply nutrients for a balanced diet.

Recommendations

- Drink a glass of Tarzan Juice (p. 222), Healthy Skin Juice (p. 222) or eat Alkaline Bomb Salad (p. 233) daily as they are strongly alkalising.
- Avoid pork with crackling, fatty beef meals and alcohol as they are highly acid-forming.
- The Eczema Diet points system will help you achieve acid–alkaline balance: your daily aim is to consume ingredients that tally to five stars ★ or more (this is coming up shortly, see the Eczema Diet points system on p. 63.)
- For a list of alkalising and acidifying foods and beverages refer to 'Eczema-safe food charts: Stage 1', p. 253.

The past 60 years of clinical research on eczema, conducted in university laboratories and by scientists, doctors and professors from all over the world, have been instrumental in showing us how our diets are intrinsically linked to skin health and the appearance of eczema. If we are to decrease the worldwide statistics of eczema and bring much-needed relief to those who are suffering, diet education is the key. Your diet not only alters how well some of your genes function, it can affect the genes you pass on to your children and their children's children. The good news is, while some genetic abnormalities are permanent, eczema is a skin disease that comes and goes, and you can prevent eczema by lovingly feeding your body to ensure it receives all the nutrients it needs for beautiful skin.

Chapter 4

The Eczema Diet: how it works

The Eczema Diet is a holistic health program that incorporates both the avoidance of offending substances and the addition of eczema-safe foods and nutrients to boost the health of your liver, blood and gastrointestinal tract, and restore skin health.

Diagram 4: How the Eczema Diet works

The Eczema Diet is designed to:

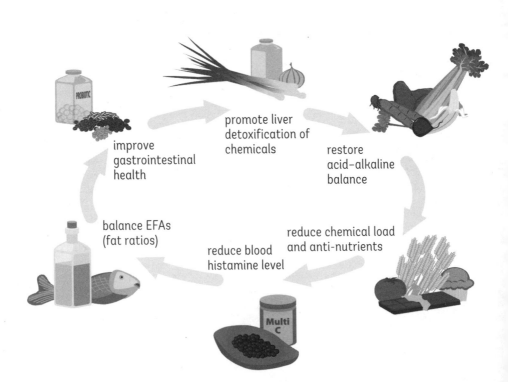

improve gastrointestinal health

promote liver detoxification of chemicals

restore acid–alkaline balance

balance EFAs (fat ratios)

reduce blood histamine level

reduce chemical load and anti-nutrients

Promote liver detoxification of chemicals

The Eczema Diet recipes supply nutrients required for Phase 2 liver detoxification and the antioxidants vitamin C, vitamin E, quercetin and alpha-lipoic acid to increase protection against free radicals, which can be created during Phase 1 liver detoxification. Promoting proper liver detoxification can reverse or reduce multiple chemical sensitivities (this can take time to achieve). While foods can supply many of the nutrients required for liver detoxification, additional supplementation is beneficial, so also refer to Table 4, 'Nutrients for liver detoxification', p. 49 and Chapter 6, 'Eczema supplements'.

Restore acid–alkaline balance

While you are on the Eczema Diet you'll learn how to create acid–alkaline balanced meals that are nutritious and beneficial for your eczema. There is a handy chart for quick reference that will help you identify alkalising and acidifying foods (see Chapter 19, 'Eczema-safe food charts', p. 252).

Reduce chemical load

The Eczema Diet consists of Stage 1 and Stage 2. These are not to be confused with Phase 1 and Phase 2 liver detoxification, which was discussed in Chapter 3. Stage 1 takes a range of problematic chemicals out of the diet to give your liver, gastrointestinal tract, kidneys and skin fewer chemicals to deal with, without suppressing liver function. This includes avoiding artificial chemicals and limiting the natural ones. Natural amines and salicylates are taken out of the diet for three days during the 3-day Alkalising Cleanse, p. 184, then they are consumed in lower amounts during Stage 1 and increased in Stage 2. During the rest of Stage 1 you can eat moderate salicylate foods such as carrots, sweet potato, cos (romaine) lettuce and beetroot, and amine-containing foods such as banana. These have been specially selected as they have the added benefit of being alkalising (beetroot is strongly alkalising) and they offer important nutrients for skin protection and maintenance.

The Eczema Diet includes non-diet information because your environment affects your skin. Exposing your skin to irritating chemicals and soap products can affect your results so it's important to have an eczema-safe skin care routine before you begin the program. Part 2 covers practical non-diet information, beginning on p. 121.

Everybody has a birthday and you might like to occasionally eat a treat or drink alcohol. The Eczema Diet covers eczema-safe party foods and special occasion treats. These foods, while containing *acid*-forming sugar, are low in chemicals that can trigger flare-ups so their occasional use should be well tolerated. (Read Chapter 15, 'Party food guide + lolly bags'.)

Reduce anti-nutrients

During Stages 1 and 2 anti-nutrients are minimised. While it is impossible to totally eliminate anti-nutrients from your diet, high intakes of anti-nutrients can be problematic for eczema sufferers because they interfere with the absorption of skin-repairing minerals.

There are two main ways anti-nutrients lower nutrients in the body. First, anti-nutrients can require a range of vitamins and minerals in order for the body to digest and detoxify them, and they rob these nutrients from your body in the process. For example, packaged foods rich in sugar and white flour are low in nutrients so while they satisfy your hunger they do not supply the nutrients your body needs for healthy skin, plus they rob some of your body's stores of vitamins and minerals during digestion and detoxification (which means fewer nutrients for skin repair and maintenance). Second, anti-nutrients can bind to nutrients so your body can't use them. For example, avidin in raw egg whites is an anti-nutrient as it binds to biotin and frequent consumption causes a deficiency (and dermatitis is the first symptom to follow). Phytic acid is another anti-nutrient that binds to the minerals calcium, iron, zinc and copper. Most types of grains and legumes, while they are an important source of dietary fibre to cleanse the bowel of toxins and cancer-causing substances, contain phytic acid. It is for this reason that I recommend soaking your grains, legumes and nuts (if consuming cashews). This is easy to do and instructions can be found in individual recipes later in the book, and discussed further in the sections 'How to soak grains', p. 80, and 'Cooking guide for legumes', p. 85.

Supply antihistamine nutrients

As eczema sufferers can have elevated histamine levels, the Eczema Diet ensures you are consuming the antihistamine nutrients vitamin C, vitamin B6 and quercetin. While these are provided in foods such as papaya, pawpaw, mung bean sprouts, brussels sprouts and spring onions (scallions), it is necessary to take vitamin C (magnesium ascorbate) and vitamin B6 in supplement form to help minimise allergic reactions and prevent histamine toxicity. Refer to Chapter 6, 'Eczema supplements'.

Balance fat ratios

The Eczema Diet shows you how to eat the correct ratios of fats by limiting omega-6 oils (no margarine and restricted use of vegetable oils) and increasing omega-3 in the diet by encouraging fish, flaxseed oil and linseed consumption. Saturated fat intake is lowered to decrease the amount of arachidonic acid you are consuming, so the omega-3 fats you consume can be more easily taken up by your cells. For more information, refer to 'Abnormal fat metabolism', p. 27.

Improve gastrointestinal health

The Eczema Diet is designed to be gentle on your gastrointestinal tract. During Stage 1, foods and drinks that can cause intestinal permeability are taken out of the diet and a probiotic supplement can be taken if desired. Once your gastrointestinal health has strengthened, you can slowly reintroduce a wider range of foods into your diet in Stage 2. If during Stage 2 you find you are still sensitive to a particular food, you should avoid it for a further 2 months and then try eating it again if desired. When reintroducing these foods, introduce one new food every 3 days so you can clearly identify problematic foods. There is an 'unofficial' Stage 3 that shows you how to introduce wheat and dairy products into your diet if you choose to consume them (p. 211). Intestinal permeability information is on p. 22 and probiotic information is on p. 113.

Symbols and abbreviations

The following is a guide to the symbols and abbreviations used throughout this book:

★	recipe or vegetable with alkalising properties
★★	recipe or vegetable with strongly alkalising properties
●	recipe or fruit rich in vitamin C and/or potassium
✴	recipe or wholegrain containing dietary fibre for gastrointestinal health
P	recipe or ingredient rich in protein and may contain iron
◆	recipe contains 1 serve of hydrating liquid
S	moderate salicylate content
SS	high to very high salicylate content
A	moderate amine content
AA	high to very high amine content
M	contains monosodium glutamate (MSG—natural or artificial flavour enhancer)
G	contains gluten
GF	gluten-free ingredient
GI	ingredient with a high glycaemic index which affects blood sugar*
Su	contains sulfites or added sulfite preservative

*If eating high GI food, take a chromium supplement once a day, or if in Stage 2 add cinnamon to the recipe to help balance blood sugar.

The Eczema Diet points system

★ ⬤ P ◆ ✳

The Eczema Diet has a simple points system to help you follow the program and meet the body's nutritional needs. Beside the name of a recipe you'll note there are a range of symbols. These are to help you quickly identify what the recipe offers you in the way of nutrition. You have five goals each day:

1. ★ ★ ★ ★ ★ Each recipe has a star rating, being no stars, one star or two stars. Your goal is to consume five or more stars each day to meet your vegetable, antioxidant and alkalising requirements for good health. This is an important step in preventing eczema.

2. ⬤ ⬤ Recipes containing fruit have an apple symbol beside them (this does not mean the recipe contains apple or that you should eat an apple). You need to consume two ⬤ each day to meet your daily vitamin C and potassium requirements. Do not eat too much fruit, especially if you have signs of fungal overgrowth, dandruff (p. 139) or *Candida albicans* (p. 23). If you are craving sweets, an extra piece of fruit is allowed.

3. ✳ ✳ Recipes containing wholegrain or wholemeal dietary fibre have beside it a 'roughage' symbol (that looks a bit like a grass prickle). You must eat at least two ✳ daily to ensure you are consuming sufficient dietary fibre to promote healthy microflora and to cleanse the bowel of toxins and carcinogens. Note that pears are a valuable source of soluble fibre so they may be marked with this symbol.

4. P P You must eat two protein P ingredients each day to ensure you are consuming enough protein for skin repair and maintenance. Protein-rich foods are usually good sources of iron, which is vital for healthy skin. If you are vegan you may require an iron supplement (refer to vegetarian and vegan information on p. 188).

5. ◆ ◆ ◆ ◆ ◆ The fifth goal is to drink plenty of liquids to hydrate the gastrointestinal tract and your skin (goal of five to a maximum of eight). Each glass of filtered water, eczema-safe vegetable juice (such as Tarzan Juice, p. 222), organic rice milk, Therapeutic Broth, p. 226, or soup counts for ◆ liquid intake.

Simple rules to follow

You can follow the Eczema Diet points system without looking at the recipes, simply by remembering the following rules:

1. Eat five serves of eczema-safe vegies daily (listed on p. 255)
2. Eat two pieces of eczema-safe fruit daily (listed on p. 256)
3. Eat at least two serves of eczema-safe grains daily (listed on p. 257)
4. Eat two serves of eczema-safe protein daily (listed on p. 258)
5. Drink five to eight glasses of filtered water daily (including eczema-safe vegetable juices and soups).

(A serve equals a ½ cup, so five serves of vegetables is approximately 2½ cups.)

For easy reference you can photocopy this page and keep it on your refrigerator. *Note:* You may choose to not follow the points system if you wish. Alternatively, you might want to follow it for the first two weeks (the menus will show you how, so you don't have to work it out by yourself). By then, you should have a good idea of how to follow the program.

Chapter 5

Top 12 eczema-safe foods + other useful ingredients

The top 12 eczema-safe foods supply valuable nutrients to help decrease inflammation and promote skin repair and maintenance. This chapter also covers general eczema-safe ingredients that you are likely to use while cooking in your kitchen, and 'The Itchy Dozen' foods that are most likely to cause flare-ups.

The top 12 eczema-safe foods are:

1. Banana A🍎

While most other fruits are acid-forming and rich in problematic chemicals, regular bananas have unique alkalising properties, thanks to their high potassium content. Bananas are salicylate-free, with the exception of sugar bananas (SS, AA) which should be avoided. Bananas are a fibre-rich and nutritious energy snack. While they contain some amines, they also supply their own amine/histamine-lowering nutrients magnesium and vitamin C so this nutrient-dense snack should not pose a problem for those who are mildly sensitive to amines. Have banana as a lunch box snack, in the Healthy Skin Smoothie (p. 223), freeze them to make iceblocks (popsicles/ice lollies) or treat yourself to sliced banana on Spelt Pancakes (p. 247).

2. Papaya A🍎

Papaya is a red fruit related to yellow pawpaw and it provides a range of carotenoids, which are potent antioxidants that can modulate gene activity to protect against inflammatory damage and tumour growth, according to clinical studies.[1] The lycopene content in papaya helps to protect the skin from sun damage (there is no lycopene in pawpaw) and both fruits are rich sources of vitamin C, the antihistamine vitamin, which can help allergy sufferers manage their symptoms. Papaya contains the digestive enzyme papain, which is used in some digestive supplements to aid protein digestion. Papain kills parasites in the gut and after antibiotic use or a bout of illness you can eat a serve of papaya daily to promote recolonisation of beneficial bacteria in the gastrointestinal tract.

Papaya is usually eaten raw, with the skin and seeds removed. The seeds contain potent antimicrobial properties and they can be eaten to flush worms out of the bowel ('flush' being the operative word as they can cause severe diarrhoea, so use with caution and do not give children papaya seeds). Eating papaya flesh does not cause any of these symptoms, although the fruit does contain a moderate amount of amines so if you are highly sensitive to amines make sure you're also taking a vitamin C, B6 and calcium supplement. If papaya is not available, use pawpaw in the recipes. Recipes include Papaya Rice Paper Rolls, p. 230; Spelt Pancakes, p. 247; Healthy Skin Smoothie, p. 223; Surprise Porridge, p. 215.

3. Broth ★★◆

A well-made broth soothes the gastrointestinal tract and provides the skin-repairing amino acid glycine, which is needed to produce connective tissue and enhances detoxification of chemicals. Broth contains collagen, calcium and magnesium and for those in poor health or suffering from a cold or flu, sipping cysteine-rich broth throughout the day can reduce mucus and offer relief. Its content of chondroitin sulfate and hyaluronan helps to lubricate joints, making broth valuable for arthritis sufferers.

A regular store-bought broth will not do, however. For a steaming cup of broth to be both a food and a 'medicine' it must be made correctly — there is a trick to extracting the nutrients from the bones and this step cannot be skipped. Broth is made by adding vegetables and bones (that have a little bit of meat, cartilage and tendons left on them) to a pot with plenty of water, and the *addition of a weak acid* causes an acid-base chemical reaction and the alkaline minerals are drawn right out of the bones (similar to when you eat an acid-forming Western diet that slowly leaches calcium from your bones). Eczema-safe acids are ascorbic acid (pure vitamin C powder) and citric acid (from the baking section of larger supermarkets).

While cooking time is extensive (a minimum of 6 hours for a nutrient-dense broth), the good news is that broth is an inexpensive meal as you can use a chicken carcass or beef bones and other bones that the local butcher usually discards or sells cheaply (not pork bones, though). Beef bones that have been roasted in the oven make for a deliciously aromatic broth. Refer to Therapeutic Broth recipe, p. 226. Vegetarians and vegans can alternatively make Alkaline Vegie Broth, p. 225.

4. Potato (white and sweet potato) ⋆

An eczema sufferer needs to avoid many foods so it's comforting to know you can enjoy a side of mashed potato and homemade potato wedges. The humble potato is a valuable staple food rich in fibre, potassium and vitamin C. One medium white potato contains a whopping 600mg of potassium, making it one of the few carbohydrate-rich foods that are alkalising. A medium-sized potato contains vitamin B6 for detoxification of chemicals such as salicylates, alpha-lipoic acid for potent antioxidant protection, and 30mg of vitamin C which is enough to stave off scurvy.

Sweet potato has a lower glycaemic index than most varieties of white potatoes, making it suitable for diabetics and those with energy problems. It is anti-inflammatory and contains some salicylates. A cup of sweet potato contains 950mg of alkalising potassium, 11,520mcg of antioxidant beta-carotene, 76mg of calcium, 54mg of magnesium and 33mg of histamine-lowering vitamin C, and 26mg of choline to guard against fatty liver conditions.

Most white potatoes have a high to medium glycaemic index, with the exception of carisma potatoes which have a low GI rating. If possible, avoid high GI desiree, sebago and pontiac (in Australia); nardine and kumara (in New Zealand). Favour carisma potatoes and potatoes with a medium GI such as new potatoes and sweet potato. Recipes include Smashed Potato, p. 239; Chickpea Casserole, p. 242; Roasted Sweet Potato Salad, p. 233; Baked Fish with Mash, p. 237; Teething Rusks, p. 224; Easy Roast Chicken, p. 240; Sunshine Soup, p. 235; New Potato and Leek Soup, p. 234.

5. Buckwheat GF ✳

Buckwheat is used as a gluten-free grain and it's actually a fruit. It's available roasted and as groats, flour, pasta and tea, and the flour can be made into pancakes or added to gluten-free muffin mixes. Unlike wheat, it's gentle on the digestive tract and rich in the potent antioxidant flavonoids rutin and quercetin. In experiments, rutin has been found to prevent capillary fragility and high blood pressure. Quercetin lowers the blood histamine level and it has a strong anti-inflammatory effect as it inhibits leukotrienes, which are produced during an eczema flare-up. While buckwheat flour is not as potent, it supplies dietary fibre and is a nutritious way to add skin-repairing nutrients into your diet. Buckwheat recipes include Buckwheat Crepes (p. 248) and Buckwheat Pasta (see 'Pasta' recipe, p. 244).

6. Mung bean sprouts ★★

Mung bean sprouts are like little alkalising 'bombs' when added to your meals as they are one of the few *strongly* alkalising foods available. They contain magnesium, vitamin K, folate, potassium and vitamin C and they are salicylate-free. Mung bean sprouts must be eaten fresh and the packet used up quickly (check use-by dates and don't buy sprouts that don't have a visible use-by date or a 'packed' date listed). And wash them thoroughly in a bowl of water before use.

Sprouting your own mung beans is easy and the recipe is below. Add them to salads and savoury dishes, and they make a healthy addition to children's snacks (kids might prefer them served without the green shells). Recipes with mung bean sprouts include Design Your Own Sandwich, p. 228; Roasted Sweet Potato Salad, p. 233; Roasted Potato Stack, p. 232; Papaya Rice Paper Rolls, p. 230; and Tarzan Juice, p. 222.

Sprouting recipe

SERVES 4; PREPARATION TIME 5 MINUTES, SOAKING TIME OVERNIGHT, RINSE AND DRAIN TWICE A DAY FOR TWO DAYS

You can use this recipe to sprout mung beans, spelt grains, barley or lentils (these are your eczema-safe choices for sprouting). If using lentils they must not be 'split' lentils as they won't sprout. Whole spelt grains are available from health food shops — they may be hard to find — and they can be used to make sprouted spelt bread. In Stage 2 you can also sprout dried green peas as they are lovely to eat when sprouted.

⅓ cup dried mung beans
wide glass jar or container
cheesecloth or mesh to cover
elastic band
filtered water

Wash the mung beans before use and remove the damaged ones that look darker or split. After rinsing them, place them into a glass jar or container. Fill the jar with lukewarm water to help soften any hard beans and cover the jar with a piece of breathable cloth or mesh and secure with an elastic band. Set aside on the kitchen bench in low light, away from direct sunlight and not in a dark cupboard. Soak them overnight.

The next morning, drain off the excess water and rinse with water. To make the rinsing process simple, keep the beans in the jar and keep the mesh on and rinse. If using cloth, remove the cloth, keep the beans in the jar, fill the jar with water and place a mesh strainer over the top and drain the water. You will need to rinse and drain twice a day for at least two days. For little mung bean sprouts *rinse and drain every 8 to 12 hours* for two to three days. Larger sprouts will take four to five days and you'll need to continue the rinsing routine so they don't dry out.

As soon as the sprouts are ready, drain any excess water, dry them and store them, wrapped in a paper towel (or something to soak up the excess moisture) in an airtight container and refrigerate them. Use them within four days for maximum freshness.

7. Oats G✹

Eczema sufferers need to start their day with a nutritious breakfast and wholegrain or rolled oats provide more dietary fibre and protein than other grain cereals. They're a source of vitamin E, zinc, potassium, iron, manganese and silica, an essential mineral for strengthening connective tissue in the skin. Oats contain soluble fibre, so when they're made into porridge it appears gluey during cooking. The fibre is valuable for gastrointestinal health, helping to lower cholesterol and cleanse pathogens and toxin-loaded bile from the bowel.

Oats contain gluten because of cross contamination, as oats are usually grown near wheat crops and processed alongside wheat. Wheat-free oats are available but often hard to find, so alternatively you can soak your oats overnight to make the gluten easier to digest and this also reduces the phytic acid content (instructions are in the individual recipes in Chapter 18, 'Recipes').

Oat recipes include Omega Muesli, p. 214; New Anzac Cookies, p. 250; and Surprise Porridge, p. 215. If you are gluten intolerant make Quinoa Porridge, p. 216, as an alternative.

8. Linseeds/flaxseeds s

Linseeds, also known as flaxseeds, are small brown seeds best known for their rich content of anti-inflammatory omega-3. The seeds are a source of phytochemicals, silica, mucilage, oleic acid, protein, vitamin E and dietary fibre, for gastrointestinal and liver health. Flaxseed oil contains more than 50 per cent omega-3 essential fatty acids.

Omega-3 is highly unstable so it's easily damaged by heat and once linseeds/ flaxseeds have been processed into oil or ground into a fine powder they can go rancid if not stored correctly. For these reasons *do not buy pre-ground linseeds/ flaxseeds or LSA* (a ground mix containing linseeds, sunflower seeds and almonds) and don't purchase flaxseed oil that has not been refrigerated in the shop. Flaxseed oil must not be heated or used for frying, and should be refrigerated at all times and used up within four weeks.

Whole or finely ground linseeds can be mixed into porridge; use whole linseeds in Omega Muesli (p. 214), or sprinkled onto Eczema-safe Fruit Salad (p. 217). Flaxseed oil can be used in recipes such as Healthy Skin Smoothie (p. 223) and in Stage 2: Omega Salad Dressing (p. 219). Below is a guide to the recommended daily amounts of linseeds:

- Children aged 1–4: ½–1 teaspoon ground linseeds daily* (¼ teaspoon flaxseed oil).
- Older children: 1–2 teaspoons daily* (½ teaspoon flaxseed oil).
- Adults: 2–4 teaspoons daily* (2–3 teaspoons flaxseed oil).

*Drink plenty of water when eating linseeds as the fibre absorbs about five times the seeds' weight.

How to grind linseeds/flaxseeds

Place whole linseeds into a coffee or seed grinder and grind them to a fine powder. Grind linseeds weekly to ensure freshness and store them in a sealed glass container in the refrigerator.

9. Red cabbage ★

Cabbage is a member of the mighty Brassica family, and it's rich in vitamin C, folate and anti-cancer indoles. But it's worth swapping to the red variety as red cabbage has double the amount of dietary fibre than regular white cabbage and it contains protective purple pigments. These pigments are caused by a group of antioxidants called anthocyanins, which are powerful flavonoids that have a skin-protective effect against UV sunlight when consumed frequently. Anthocyanins help to protect blood vessels from oxidative damage, and their anti-inflammatory properties activate the production of collagen for healthy skin. Anthocyanins also have to ability to block glycation and AGE formation (advanced glycation end products), which degrade collagen and elastic fibres in the skin and play a role in skin ageing.

It is recommended to steam or stir-fry cabbage as cooking deactivates the goitrins (which can affect the thyroid). Eat red cabbage about three times a week. You can add it to recipes including Baked Fish with Mash, p. 237; Easy Roast Chicken, p. 240; and My Favourite Lamb Cutlets, p. 243, or add red cabbage to any meal where you are steaming or stir-frying vegetables.

10. Spring onions ★

Spring onions, also referred to as scallions and shallots, are part of the onion family, and like the onion, spring onions contain histamine-lowering, anti-inflammatory quercetin. Like garlic (but in lower concentrations) spring onions possess antioxidant flavonoids that convert to allicin when cut or crushed. Lab experiments show that allicin helps liver cells to reduce cholesterol and has antibacterial, anti-viral and anti-fungal properties. Spring onions contain folate, vitamin C, beta-carotene and lutein and are one of the richest sources of vitamin K, which is vital for healthy skin. Just 50g of raw spring onions provides 103mcg of vitamin K, nearly double the daily adequate intake for adults. Recipes include Chickpea Rice, p. 231; Country Chicken Soup, p. 236; Sticks and Stones, p. 238.

11. Fish P

High fish intake during pregnancy is associated with a decreased risk of eczema and fish is a good source of protein, vitamin D and iodine.[2,3] Studies show two to three serves of fish each week are beneficial for elevating mood and increasing the health of the brain, skin and heart. Good sources of omega-3, EPA and DHA include trout, salmon, sardines, herring and fish oil supplements. Other minor sources of EPA and

DHA include low-fat seafood such as carp, pike, haddock, oysters, clams, scallops and squid. It's important to favour eczema-safe fish, which are low in mercury.

Safe seafood

The following seafoods are low in mercury, as is the case with all small-sized fish (if in doubt ask your local fishmonger at the fish shop). The general rule is: the higher up the food chain and the bigger the fish (e.g. shark/flake), the more mercury it may contain.

- trout and rainbow trout (AA)
- flathead
- dory (small fillets)
- hake
- bream
- shrimp
- flounder
- herring
- sardines (AA)
- lobster
- oysters
- quality canned tuna in springwater/brine* (AA)
- salmon (AA)

*You can make a healthy snack with 95g (3½ oz) of canned tuna once a week, as canned tuna is sourced from smaller sized tuna.

AA = rich in amines (not to be confused with arachidonic acid, which is also abbreviated to AA). Do not consume amine-rich fish more than once a week and discontinue use if you have an adverse reaction.

Fish to avoid

The following fish contain high levels of mercury and should be avoided. Health authorities recommend if you eat a serve of mercury-rich fish you should then avoid eating all seafood for at least two weeks afterwards to allow time for your mercury levels to reduce.

- flake/shark (often used for fish and chips)

- large snapper
- swordfish
- marlin
- king mackerel
- perch (orange roughy)
- barramundi (larger fillets)
- gemfish
- large ling
- larger tuna (albacore, southern bluefin)

Do not eat frozen fish as this is ten times higher in histamines. Avoid prawns as they are treated with sulfite preservative (cooked prawns and shrimp may be preservative-free but you will need to check). While you have eczema, avoid smoked salmon and other smoked fish as they are highly acidifying and may contain chemicals and increased amines.

Salmon and trout are commonly farmed in Western countries such as Australia and it has been suggested that these fish contain less nutrients than fish fresh from the ocean. If you cannot buy ocean-caught fish, farmed fish is an acceptable source.

Both adults and children can eat low-mercury fish *twice a week*, the portion being no bigger than the palm of your hand. Do not eat seafood more than three times a week because over-consumption of seafood may eventually lead to mercury accumulation. Recipes include Sticks and Stones, p. 238; Roasted Potato Stack, p. 232; Baked Fish with Mash, p. 237.

12. Beetroot ★ ★ s

Beetroot is an important vegetable for eczema sufferers as it has strong alkalising properties which boost liver detoxification of salicylates and other chemicals. It contains moderate salicylates, and it's abundant in antioxidants, folic acid and iron. Beetroot is a potent blood cleanser and research shows that beetroot consumption lowers blood pressure and has an aspirin-like effect, reducing the risk of blood clots.

Grate fresh, peeled beetroot into salads or salad sandwiches and use beetroot in freshly made vegetable juices. Do not consume canned beetroot as it contains vinegar. Recipes include Healthy Skin Juice, p. 222; Design Your Own Sandwich, p. 228; and you can add grated beetroot to Alkaline Bomb Salad, p. 233.

Other useful ingredients

While they didn't quite make the top 12, the following are some other useful ingredients for those with eczema.

Lecithin granules

Lecithin is a phospholipid made up of essential fatty acids, phosphorous, inositol and choline, which is an important component of bile, a substance the liver makes to remove unwanted chemicals and fats from the body. Lecithin helps the body to utilise fats correctly (making it ideal for eczema sufferers with abnormal fat metabolism); it's essential for liver function and helps to lower cholesterol. A healthy body produces small amounts of lecithin and it is present in protein foods such as meats, fish, soy and eggs. High-fat diets increase the need for lecithin and if you don't consume enough lecithin, fatty liver can result.

Store-bought lecithin granules, made from soy, look like tiny yellow beads and have a pleasant malty flavour. Egg lecithin is available but it contains predominantly saturated fat and eczema sufferers are more likely to be allergic to eggs so this form is not recommended. A tablespoon of lecithin granules makes a great addition to smoothies with added flaxseed oil, as the lecithin helps your body utilise the omega-3 essential fatty acids from the oil (I highly recommend you consume flaxseed oil with the addition of lecithin). Soy lecithin-containing recipes include Omega Muesli, p. 214 Healthy Skin Smoothie, p. 223; and the Stage 2 recipe Flaxseed Lemon Drink, p. 223.

Age range	Soy lecithin granule dosages*
Adults	1 tablespoon (8g) daily with food (supplies approx. 250mg of choline)
14–18 years	3 teaspoons (6g) daily with food (supplies approx. 187mg of choline)
9–13 years	2 teaspoons (4g) daily with food (supplies approx. 125mg of choline)
4–8 years	1 teaspoon (2g) daily with food (supplies approx. 62mg choline)
1–3 years	½ teaspoon (1g) daily with food (supplies approx. 31mg of choline)
0–12 months	choline is supplied in breastmilk (especially when the mother's health and diet is good), infant formula and infant food if on solids

*Don't consume genetically modified soy lecithin (favour GMO-free soy) and do not consume soy lecithin if you are allergic to soy.

Cooking oil: rice bran oil

Rice bran oil is low in salicylates and, like olive oil, rice bran oil contains oleic acid and vitamin E. It contains omega-6 essential fatty acids which should only be consumed in moderation. Rice bran oil also has a high smoking point.

When choosing an oil for frying at high heat it's important to consider the smoking point — the temperature at which the oil begins to break down and produce smoke. A smoking oil is a sign damage is occurring, the nutrients are being destroyed and the oil is fast becoming bad for your health (at this point you should carefully pour off the oil (if possible), wipe the pan clean and start again. To reduce the risk of burnt oil, you want to use a cooking oil that has a high smoking point. A basic rule is, the more 'extra virgin' or unrefined an oil is, the more easily it will burn. There are some exceptions to this rule and rice bran oil is one of them as it is relatively heat stable and its high smoking point makes rice bran oil an excellent choice for baking and frying.

Cooking oil	Smoking point °C	Smoking point °F
refined safflower oil	266°C	510°F
rice bran oil	254°C	490°F
ghee (Indian clarified dairy butter)	252°C	485°F
refined/light olive oil	242°C	468°F
refined soybean oil	238°C	460°F
refined coconut oil	232°C	450°F
refined canola oil	204°C	400°F
extra virgin olive oil	190°C	375°F
extra virgin coconut oil	177°C	350°F
butter	121–149°C	250–300°F
virgin safflower oil	107°C	225°F

Note: The oils shaded in grey are eczema-safe and suitable for use during Stage 1 of the Eczema Diet.

Cooking oil recommendations

- While you have eczema, do not cook with olive oil, coconut oil, canola oil or any other oil that is not on the Eczema-safe shopping guides, pp. 260–263.
- Rice bran oil can burn on very high heat so turn down your frying pan to medium once it has heated up.
- Rice bran oil contains omega-6 so it should only be used sparingly.
- While you have eczema a cooking oil-free diet would be the healthiest choice (this means using no cooking oil, not even rice bran oil). This may be difficult to achieve so alternatively see if you can have some 'oil-free' days (on these days, make salads or one of the soup recipes or steam vegies and have them with boiled or steamed chicken or steamed fish).

Sweetener: rice malt syrup

Ideally, your diet should have no added sweeteners, but for those of you who wish to use sweetener the best choice is rice malt syrup for two reasons: it is alkalising (whereas all other sweeteners convert to acid in the body), and it's low in salicylates and other chemicals. Rice malt syrup is milder than honey so more may be required in recipes.

In order of preference, here are the sweeteners eczema sufferers can use in recipes:

- rice malt syrup (alkalising, low in chemicals)
- real maple syrup (acid-producing, low in chemicals)
- golden syrup* (acid-producing, low in chemicals)

*A couple of the sweet recipes require golden syrup, which is a less refined sugar syrup. If this ingredient is not available in your country use real maple syrup instead — do not use imitation maple syrup as it may contain additives.

Barley malt is often used to sweeten soy milks and this sweetener should be eczema-safe if you are not gluten intolerant. It you're allergic to gluten use *malt-free* soy milk or organic rice milk as they are both gluten-free.

Sweeteners to avoid

If you have chronic candida or fungal overgrowth then I recommend you go sweetener-free. Sugar is strongly acid-producing and should only be used, for example, on rare occasions when you make birthday cake. For those of you who have a child with eczema, I don't recommend you suddenly take every sugary food out of their diet. You can offer them sweet eczema-safe alternatives such as New Anzac Cookies, p. 250 and Pear Muffins, p. 249.

In general, it's important that eczema sufferers avoid the following sweeteners as they may worsen eczema symptoms:

- honey
- molasses
- fructose
- stevia
- artificial sweeteners (all kinds, listed on p. 35)
- refined, white sugar (highly acid producing).

Sugar cravings

It's important to listen to your sugar cravings as your body may be telling you something important about your diet. Before you reach for a biscuit or a chocolate, however, consider the following: sugar cravings can be a sign your body is craving vitamin C or potassium from sweet fruits, or magnesium and chromium from quality carbohydrate grains. Give your body the nutrients it craves: eat papaya or pawpaw to boost your vitamin C, eat banana for potassium and take a supplement containing magnesium and chromium — and watch your cravings disappear.

Non-dairy milks

Dairy products, especially animal milks (cow, goat, sheep), are not suitable for eczema sufferers. It is possible to follow this diet without any milk substitutes and alternatively eat protein twice a day and consume five serves of alkalising vegetables for bone health (an alkalising diet is better at strengthening bones than dairy products). For those of you who would like to consume milk in your porridge, smoothies and baked goods, here are the best options for you:

Organic soy milk G

Like all processed food products, soy milk has its good and bad points and there are different qualities available. The best choice is any variety containing organic 'whole' soybeans as these are less processed and of the highest quality. Do not buy soy milk listing 'soy isolate' in the ingredients, as soy isolate was once considered a waste product and may contain aluminium. The ingredient barley malt, which is added to soy milks for added sweetness, contains gluten so if you are gluten intolerant look for 'malt-free' soy milk or use organic rice milk. If you choose to drink soy milk or any milk keep in mind they are processed products so consume only in moderation (e.g. a splash on your porridge or to make creamy Smashed Potato, p. 239).

If available, choose organic soy milk that is fresh (in the refrigerated section of the supermarket), and one that contains added fibre and calcium and has a low glycaemic index.

Rice milk GF

If you choose to drink milk, rice milk is a sweet, watery milk that is low allergy and low in chemicals so it is regarded as eczema-safe. If purchasing rice milk, favour organic rice milk that is 'calcium fortified', which means it has added calcium. Rice milk often contains sunflower oil, which is usually eczema-safe. Although naturopaths tend to favour rice milk over soy milk, be aware that rice milk has a very high glycaemic index so it's not suitable for diabetics or those with hypoglycaemia or energy problems of any kind. For this reason, only use rice milk in moderation and take a chromium supplement daily to promote blood sugar balance (for chromium information see p. 104).

Oat milk G

A serve of oat milk is rich in fibre, calcium, vitamin A and if you are vegan it is a valuable source of iron (it contains 10 per cent of the recommended dietary intake). Oat milk is lactose-free and it contains gluten so don't use oat milk if you are allergic to wheat or gluten.

What about almond milk?

Almond milk is rich in salicylates and may cause flare-ups so it not suitable for eczema sufferers.

Eczema-safe grains ⁕

The following grains are eczema-safe because they are low in natural chemicals and contain no artificial additives. If possible, soak grains before consuming them.

- spelt (G)
- buckwheat (GF)
- brown rice (not instant) (GI)(GF)
- basmati rice (GF)
- quinoa (not puffed) (GI)(GF)
- wholegrain or rolled oats (porridge) (G)
- oat bran (G)
- rice bran (GF)
- barley (G)
- rye (G)

Which grains did not make the list?

The Eczema Diet is wheat-free. Going wheat-free for a few months gives the digestive tract time to repair and you might find that you are better able to tolerate wheat after having a break from it. The Eczema Diet is not gluten-free but if you are gluten intolerant it's easy to adapt this diet by avoiding all gluten-containing products including wheat, spelt, rye, barley and oats (denoted with a 'G' in the recipes).

Also avoid corn, polenta (cornmeal) and most commercial breakfast cereals while you have eczema as they are rich in irritating chemicals such as salicylates.

Amaranth, millet, tapioca, jasmine rice, instant/quick-cooking rice and Japanese glutinous rice did not make the list because they have an incredibly high GI, which triggers high insulin in the blood (refer to Diagram 3, 'How prostaglandins control inflammation', p. 30, for reasons why high insulin is bad for eczema).

Why soak your grains?

Grains, legumes and nuts contain phytic acid, an anti-nutrient that reduces the absorption of zinc, copper, calcium and iron. Traditional methods of making sourdough bread, such as fermenting, sprouting and soaking, reduce the phytic acid content, increase gluten tolerance and make minerals more available for skin repair and maintenance. While consuming grains, legumes and nuts in moderation should not cause deficiencies there is an increased risk when large quantities are consumed.

Soaking grains is optional during the Eczema Diet but it is highly recommended, it's easy and it can quickly become a habit. The key is to think ahead and always have a couple of bowls of soaking grains on your kitchen bench. If the bench is bare, you know it's time to soak some more grains (see 'How to soak grains', below).

Soaking acids

Using a weak acid when soaking grains is an optional step but it is highly recommended as it changes the pH of the water, speeding up the breakdown of phytic acid and this increases the nutritional content of the grains. Weak acids suitable for eczema sufferers are ascorbic acid (pure vitamin C powder) and citric acid. Ascorbic acid is preferable and is available online and from compounding chemists. Do not use other types of vitamin C. Citric acid is usually found in the baking section in larger supermarkets. Although rare, it's possible to be sensitive to citric acid so if gastrointestinal disturbances occur, discontinue use. Ascorbic acid and citric acid add a lovely tangy flavour to dips and spreads (see Sesame-free Hummus, p. 220; Parsley Pesto, p. 221), and they can be used to make Therapeutic Broth, p. 226.

How to soak grains

Grains are generally soaked overnight for use in the morning or soaked first thing in the morning if you are consuming the grains in the evening. The exceptions are barley and buckwheat which need less than 2 hours soaking time. When soaking grains you will need:

- a bowl or glass container
- grains of choice (see Table 7, 'Grain soaking and cooking times', p. 81)
- filtered water (at room temperature or tepid)
- a clean tea towel or plastic wrap (to keep out potential bugs)
- a pinch of ascorbic acid or citric acid (optional).

Place your choice of grain into a bowl and cover with double the quantity of water. Then mix in a pinch of ascorbic acid or citric acid and cover with plastic wrap or a clean tea towel. Leave on the bench away from direct sunlight (do not refrigerate or place in a dark cupboard). Soak for the recommended length of time (see Table 7). Then drain off the water using a strainer, rinse with fresh water to remove the vitamin C or citric acid flavour, and the grains are ready to use (see Table 7 for approximate cooking times). Use soaked grains within 13 hours or strain, rinse and refrigerate them until needed (use refrigerated grains within 3 days).

Table 7: Grain soaking and cooking times

Grain	Raw quantity	Soaking time	Cooking time
buckwheat, whole	½ cup per adult	at least 1 hour	10 minutes (refer to packaging)
barley (G)	1 cup (½ cup in Country Chicken Soup, p. 236)	at least 2 hours	20 minutes if soaked, 45 minutes if unsoaked
rolled (porridge) oats (G)	½ cup per adult ⅓ cup per child ¼ cup per toddler	12 hours/overnight	Omega Muesli, p. 214: no cooking required porridge: 15 minutes
quinoa (not puffed)	½ cup per adult ⅓ cup per child ¼ cup per toddler	12 hours/overnight	20 minutes+
basmati rice, white rice	1½ cups*	12 hours/overnight	7–10 minutes
brown rice	2½ cups*	12 hours/overnight	20–25 minutes

*Quantities are enough to feed a family of four.

Eczema-safe bread

Eczema-safe breads are generally easy to digest (or gentler on the digestive tract than wheat breads). If you can eat gluten then spelt bread is the top choice for eczema sufferers. Spelt bread tastes similar to wheat and spelt sourdough bread uses the traditional, non-yeast method of breadmaking, making it naturally lower in phytic acid and low GI (so it supplies energy slowly and does not trigger high blood insulin). Spelt recipes include Spelt Lavash Bread (flat bread or baked into spelt chips), p. 229; Spelt Pancakes, p. 247; and Pear Muffins, p. 249.

When choosing gluten-free bread refer to the eczema-safe grain and flour lists on p. 81 and below. If buying store-bought breads, avoid artificial preservative 282 (calcium propionate).

Eczema-safe breads include:

- spelt sourdough bread
- gluten-free bread (if necessary)
- plain sprouted breads (may contain gluten)
- rye bread (no wheat)
- Spelt Lavash Bread (flat bread), p. 229
- sprouted spelt loaf.

Eczema-safe flour

Baking with spelt flour is preferable as the gluten makes the recipes work brilliantly, and the kids can't tell the difference. Buckwheat makes a very nutritious flour but it is an acquired taste, best used in pancakes with rice malt syrup and sliced banana. If you need to use a packet of gluten-free flour check for additives (see Table 3, 'Additives to avoid', p. 34) and note that highly processed white cornflour is acceptable to consume in small amounts but corn or yellow maize are not eczema-safe. As flours are highly processed or ground into a fine powder, making them fast to digest, they usually have a high GI rating. If the flour is used in nutritious recipes containing protein, the GI may be reduced.

The Eczema Diet recipes do not use all the following flours; the ones used in the recipes are the first three flours:

- buckwheat flour (GF)
- rice flour/brown rice flour (GI)(GF)
- spelt flour (wholemeal if available) (G)
- oat flour (G)
- quinoa flour (GI)(GF)
- arrowroot flour (GF).

If you are looking for baking helpers, use gluten-free baking powder or bicarbonate of soda (baking soda, also gluten-free).

Animal and vegetarian protein ᴘ

Your skin, muscles, brain cells, hair and nails need protein to function; without it your muscles would begin to waste, your skin, hair and nails would suffer and your body would swell with fluid retention (and children stop growing without protein). On the other hand, if you eat *too much* protein — for example, if you follow a high-protein low-carb diet for too long — you can end up with muscle wasting, constipation and an increased risk of bowel cancer, skin rashes, acne and/or kidney problems. Therefore, for optimal health of the skin and body, a balanced or moderate amount of protein is needed in the diet.

Eczema-safe protein

Here are some guidelines for choosing eczema-safe protein:

- Protein from animal sources should be free range or organic where possible.
- It's essential to remove chicken skin and cut fatty pieces off meats.
- Buy only the freshest cuts of meat which are free of preservatives and low in fat.
- If buying mince, ask your butcher to grind it fresh as most packaged mince (and packaged fish) contains preservatives.
- Don't consume meat or fish that has a strong or unpleasant odour.
- Don't consume fish that has been frozen as they are rich in amines.

Choose from the following animal and vegetable protein sources:

- turkey
- lamb
- veal
- trout/rainbow trout (AA)
- white fish, fresh (eczema-safe fish, p. 72)
- canned salmon or tuna in springwater/brine (AA)
- preservative-free mince (lamb, chicken, veal)

- canned or dried beans (not broad beans)
- green beans
- mung bean sprouts
- lentil sprouts
- lentils

Raw egg whites

To avoid egg white injury (p. 96), it is imperative that you avoid consuming products containing hidden sources of raw egg white, including:

- whole-egg mayonnaise
- some creamy salad dressings/coleslaw dressing
- raw cake/pancake mix
- some commercial dips including baba ganoush and tuna dip
- hollandaise sauce
- powdered egg protein shakes
- traditional chocolate mousse
- icing on traditional wedding cake
- pavlova.

Protein foods to avoid

If you suffer from eczema it is best to avoid the following protein foods:

- deli meats such as salami, bacon and ham (which contain nitrates)
- sliced/processed chicken and turkey (contain flavour enhancers)
- sausages (nitrates)
- pork, bacon, ham and beef (strongly acid-forming)
- liver (rich in pesticides and vitamin A)
- frozen fish (rich in histamines)
- frozen meats and leftovers (can be high in amines)
- prawns (they are treated with sulfite preservative)
- tempeh
- vegan patties/sausages (additives, flavour enhancers and/or salicylates)
- eggs, if an allergy or intolerance is suspected*
- all dairy products.

*As eczema sufferers are often highly allergic to eggs, I suggest all eczema sufferers avoid eating eggs during Stage 1 of the Eczema Diet even if no allergy is suspected. Then during Stage 2, after your eczema has cleared up, if you are not allergic to eggs, you may like to add them to your diet.

How much protein?

Ensure you consume some sort of protein every day — preferably in two of your main meals. Between 45g (1½oz) and 100g (3½oz) of cooked meat such as chicken will provide adults with sufficient daily protein, as will two small lean lamb chops, two slices of roast meat or half a chicken breast fillet. An 80–120g serve (2½–4½oz) of fish will also give you enough protein for the day.

If you're vegetarian or vegan, have two serves of vegetarian protein each day alongside a grain such as brown rice, as this makes the protein more 'complete'. One cup of lentils, green beans, chickpeas (garbanzo beans), split peas or kidney beans served with wholegrain carbohydrates will provide your daily protein needs. Aim for two small serves of protein in your daily diet; children and pregnant women should have two or three serves.

Cooking guide for legumes P

Legumes are rich in magnesium and potassium and supply dietary fibre, protein and slow-release carbohydrate for energy. Canned legumes such as brown lentils, chickpeas (garbanzo beans) and mixed beans are a convenient option. However, some nutrients are destroyed during the canning process and some cans are coated with bisphenol A (BPA) which can leach into the canned food (the Food Standards Agency in the United Kingdom says that BPA is known to have 'weak oestrogenic effects' and it could disrupt hormone systems, although more research is warranted). If using canned legumes, it's also essential to drain and *thoroughly rinse* them as they are packed with a fair amount of salt. Dried legumes which are home-cooked are the best and most nutritious choice. Here is your guide for cooking legumes:

Step 1: Rinsing and sorting
Whether using canned or dried legumes, it's important to rinse the legumes and pick out any discoloured or shrivelled legumes or small stones.

Step 2: Soaking dried legumes

Most dried legumes should be soaked overnight in water; this helps to reduce phytic acid, promote even cooking and reduce simmering time. For every 1 cup of legumes use 4 cups of water.

Long soak method: Place legumes and water in a saucepan, cover and soak overnight at room temperature (8+ hours). In the morning, discard the water and use new water for cooking.

Quick soak method: Boil the legumes in water for 5 minutes and then remove from heat, cover and soak for 2 hours. Discard the water. Then add fresh water for cooking (refer to Step 3).

If you have flatulence problems when eating beans, combine both methods: bring a large saucepan of water to the boil then add the legumes and boil for 2 minutes. Remove from heat, cover and soak overnight. Important: discard the soaked water as it contains the indigestible sugars that promote gas.

Step 3: Cooking legumes

After soaking the legumes (if required — see below), add the necessary amount of water (4 cups of water for every 1 cup of legumes is ideal). Avoid stirring the beans while cooking as it can damage them. Do not add salt as it can toughen the beans if added too early.

Lentils are quick to cook, but for all other beans check their progress after 45 minutes with this simple test: if the legumes are cooked they should be soft enough to easily mash using the back of a fork. All cooking times are approximate and will vary depending on how long it has been since they were harvested.

What types of dried legumes do not need soaking?

Dried lentils (red and brown/green), split peas (green and yellow) and black-eyed peas do not need to be soaked. Adzuki and mung beans only need to be soaked for 1 to 2 hours. However, make sure you rinse these beans and lentils thoroughly, changing the water two or three times until it runs clear.

Table 8: Legume cooking times

Legume	Approximate cooking times
adzuki beans	45 minutes–1½ hours
black-eyed peas/beans	1–2 hours
cannellini beans	1 hour
chickpeas (garbanzo beans)	1½–2 hours (allow to cool in cooking water)
dried split peas	up to 45 minutes
kidney beans	1 hour+
lentils	20–30 minutes
lima beans	1–2 hours
mung beans	45–60 minutes
navy beans	1–2 hours
pinto beans	1–2 hours

Note: 1 cup of legumes usually makes 2½ cups when cooked.

How much food should go on your plate?
★ ● P ◆ ✳

A simple rule when serving lunch and dinner is this: fill half your plate with vegetables, one quarter with quality protein (meat, fish, beans) and the other quarter with quality carbohydrates (rice, quinoa, spelt bread). If you want dessert, favour eczema-safe fruits such as banana, papaya, pawpaw or pear. These rules also apply to

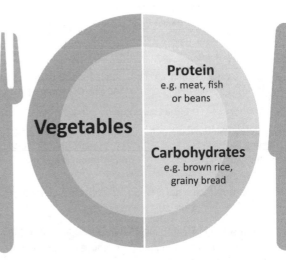

children; just use appropriate child-sized plates and read 'protein' information on portion sizes.

Salt

Commercial table salt is not eczema-safe as it can have an added anti-caking agent containing aluminium, most of the nutritious minerals have been removed and it's acid-producing so it can disrupt the body's acid–alkaline balance. If you'd like to use salt buy quality iodised rock salt, as iodine is important for the skin, or Celtic or macro sea salt — eczema-safe salt should be grey in colour, indicating it's unprocessed and mineral-rich, and it should not contain anti-caking agent. These alkaline salts are okay to use in moderation. Do not add salt to your food if you have high blood pressure.

Table 9: Choosing eczema-safe alternatives

Foods to avoid	Eczema-safe alternatives
dairy products, cow/goat/sheep milk, milkshakes	organic rice milk, oat milk, organic soy milk (not 'soy isolate') in moderation
margarine, dairy-free margarine, softened butter (contains additives/oils), jams, spreads	Sesame-free Hummus, p. 220; Bean Dip, p. 219; Banana Carob Spread, p. 220; (Stage 2: pure organic butter or ghee if no allergy to dairy)
pork, ham, bacon, beef, deli meats, sausages, mince with preservatives (not listed on packaging)	lean lamb, free-range chicken, beef bones used in broth, lean lamb/veal/chicken mince (ask butcher for additive-free or freshly made mince)
smoked salmon/fish, canned tuna in oil or olive oil	baked or grilled trout or smaller white fish (see fish information p. 72)
raw egg white, whole-egg mayonnaise, dips with egg	egg replacer (baking section), Sesame-free Hummus, p. 220, instead of mayonnaise (Stage 2: free-range egg, cooked, 1–2 eggs a week maximum, if not allergic to egg)
most fruits (rich in natural chemicals), fruit juices	peeled pear, banana (not sugar variety), papaya
tomato, tomato-containing products, capsicum (pepper), mushrooms, pumpkin (winter squash), broccoli	carrot, celery, potato, sweet potato, green beans, brussels sprouts, cabbage (white and red)
dark leafy greens, spinach, silver beet, rocket (arugula) etc. (in Stage 1 of diet)	cos (romaine) lettuce, iceberg lettuce

Foods to avoid	Eczema-safe alternatives
most herbs and spices (in Stage 1 of diet)	parsley (in moderation), parsley flakes, chives
onions, most sprouts	leeks, spring onion/scallion/shallot, garlic, dried garlic powder, mung bean sprouts, lentil sprouts, sprouted spelt
avocado	Sesame-free Hummus, p. 220; Bean Dip, p. 219
soy sauce/tamari, tomato sauce, barbecue sauce and other sauces, salad dressings of any kind	Sesame-free Hummus, p. 220; Parsley Pesto, p. 221; Omega Salad Dressing, p. 219 (Stage 2 only)
dried fruits	peeled pear, papaya, pawpaw, banana, Baked Banana Chips, p. 218
nuts	unsalted raw cashews (if no allergy to nuts; do not have roasted)
vinegar (all types), pickled foods, gherkins	(Stage 2 only: quality apple cider vinegar if no allergy to sulfites)
olive oil, canola oil, coconut oil, vegetable oils	rice bran oil
wheat products, wheat flour, plain flour, wheat bread, commercial wheat breakfast cereals, wheat pasta	spelt flour, spelt sourdough, buckwheat, brown rice, basmati rice, quinoa, rolled (porridge) oats, wheat-free oats, rice bran, brown rice flour/rice flour, barley, rye, potato flour, soy flour, rye flour, plain gluten-free bread (no corn/maize), gluten-free rice pasta, buckwheat pasta
corn, cornflakes, cornflour (cornstarch), corn chips	quinoa porridge, rolled oat porridge, puffed rice cereal (preferably brown), (occasional use of white cornflour e.g. in gluten-free baking is acceptable), plain rice crackers (no additives)
broad beans	other beans, kidney beans, navy beans, lentils, cannellini beans, chickpeas (garbanzo beans), green beans
sugar, honey, molasses, artificial sweeteners, cocoa powder	rice malt syrup, real maple syrup, golden syrup (used only in baking), carob powder, real vanilla essence
soft drink (sodas), diet soft drink, flavoured mineral water	filtered water, natural springwater (not carbonated)
tap water	filtered water, natural spring water (not carbonated)
coffee, tea, herbal tea (all kinds), fruit juice	Therapeutic Broth, p. 226; Tarzan Juice, p. 222; Healthy Skin Juice, p. 222; Healthy Skin Smoothie, p. 223; Choco Milk, p. 245
biscuits, muffins, snack foods, cakes, pastries, chips, pancake mix, confectionery/lollies/candy, chocolate	Pear Muffins, p. 249; Spelt Pancakes, p. 247; Buckwheat Crepes, p. 248; plain rice crackers/cakes (no additives) with Banana Carob Spread, p. 220; carrot and celery sticks; Baked Banana Chips, p. 218; New Anzac Cookies, p. 250 (occasional consumption only)

See the Eczema-safe shopping guides on pp. 259–263 for a complete list of eczema-safe items.

The itchy dozen

Not counting allergy foods, here are the general foods and beverages most likely to give you itchy skin or cause your eczema to flare up:

1. cow's milk and other dairy products
2. grapes (including wines, sultanas, raisins and grape-containing juices)
3. oranges (and orange juice)
4. kiwi fruit
5. soy sauce/tamari sauce
6. tomato and products containing tomato
7. avocado
8. dark green vegetables (broccoli, spinach, silver beet, wheatgrass juice etc.)
9. dried fruits (apricots, dates, figs etc.)
10. deli meats (sausages, ham, bacon, meats with flavour enhancers etc.)
11. corn and products containing corn
12. junk food, especially coloured lollies and sweets.

Chapter 6

Eczema supplements

A range of nutrients work together to repair, renew and moisturise your skin. These are covered in detail in this chapter.

Note: For best results these nutrients need to be used in conjunction with the Eczema Diet. The following supplements should not be combined with herbal preparations or supplements containing vegetable extracts such as broccoli as they are rich in salicylates and other plant chemicals.

Vitamin C

The body is truly remarkable and resourceful. It makes many of its own vitamins in the gastrointestinal tract and it stores minerals in the liver and bones; however, the body does not store or manufacture vitamin C so it must be consumed in your diet. Vitamin C (also known as ascorbic acid) aids the absorption of iron and copper, it's vital for the formation of collagen in the skin, guards against infections and is required for liver detoxification. Vitamin C is a natural antihistamine as it destroys the imidazole ring of the histamine molecule.[1] For this reason it's imperative that allergy sufferers avoid developing vitamin C deficiency as it can result in histamine toxicity and allergic reactions may increase in severity. You can prevent this from occurring by eating vitamin C-rich papaya, pawpaw or brussels sprouts and by taking a vitamin C supplement.

Signs of vitamin C deficiency include allergies, dry skin, bumpy/rough skin, easy bruising, small purplish spots on skin, fatigue, depression, tooth loss, haemorrhaging, bleeding gums, swelling of lower extremities, joint pain (mimics arthritis) and poor wound healing.[2,3] In infants, low or no intake of vitamin C (from breastmilk, when the mother is vitamin C deficient) can mimic 'shaken baby syndrome' (easy bruising, brain haemorrhage, blood pooling in the eyes and fractures).[4] According to recent research, Americans continue to suffer from scurvy (the 'sailor's disease' of the 1700s) because people aren't eating enough fruits and vegetables.[5]

Vitamin C deficiency can occur from dieting, from following a no-fruit diet (such as high-protein, low-carb diets), vaccinations/immunisations, frequent aspirin intake or high salicylate ingestion, the birth control pill, stress, cigarette smoking and diabetes.[6,7] Not all fruits and vegetables contain adequate vitamin C.

Food sources of vitamin C

The following is a list of food sources of vitamin C with the content of vitamin C listed in milligrams:

- 100g (3½oz) brussels sprouts, 110mg
- 150g (5oz) papaya/pawpaw, 90mg
- 100g (3½oz) cabbage, 45mg
- 100g (3½oz) leek, 30mg
- 100g (3½oz) sweet potato, 25mg
- 100g (3½oz) swede (rutabaga)/turnip, 25mg
- 1 medium potato, 30mg
- 100g (3½oz) green beans, 20mg
- 1 banana, 15mg
- 3 spring onions (scallions), 15mg
- 10g (⅓oz) parsley, 10mg
- 100g (3½oz) guava, 245mg (not suitable during Stage 1).

Vitamin C dosages for eczema sufferers	
Age range	Vitamin C total daily intake* (supplement dosages in brackets)
Adults	200–500mg (80mg in supplement form taken with food) and consume 2½ cups fruit and vegetables, supplying approx. 200mg vitamin C
5–17 years	70–120mg (40mg in supplement form, taken with food) and consume 1½ cups fruit and vegetables
1–4 years	60–100mg (20mg in supplement form, taken with food) and consume 1 cup fruit and vegetables
0–12 months	25–35mg from breastmilk or formula. Also give infants on solids 1 tablespoon to ½ cup of fruit and vegetables daily, depending on age and appetite.

Dosage note

Total daily intake is the minimum to maximum recommended amount obtained daily from both foods and a supplement. If a supplement is recommended, the individual supplement dosages and instructions are listed in brackets. For example, for adults the minimum amount of vitamin C from both foods and supplement is 200mg and the maximum is 500mg. Ascorbic acid is acidic so choose a buffered 'ascorbate' form of vitamin C such as magnesium ascorbate, calcium ascorbate or sodium ascorbate.

To meet your daily requirement for vitamin C (in amounts that are adequate for preventing histamine toxicity), vitamin C-rich fruits and vegetables must be eaten daily. For example, eat sliced papaya on porridge in the morning, a side salad with lunch and green beans and brussels sprouts with dinner.

Caution

Do not chew vitamin C tablets as they can wear away teeth enamel, making teeth sensitive and painful. A powdered multi-formula supplement is preferable or a solid tablet swallowed whole (for children use a powdered supplement to avoid choking).

Vitamin C thins the blood. Do not take vitamin C supplements if you have haemochromatosis or if you have been prescribed aspirin, anticoagulants or antidepressants.

Powerful co-nutrients

- Vitamin C + vitamin B3 (delta-5-desaturase enzyme reactions/FADS1 gene).
- Vitamin C + glycine (collagen formation and liver detoxification).
- Vitamin C + quercetin + vitamin B6 (natural antihistamines).

Glycine

Glycine is an amino acid found in protein and it's beneficial for eczema sufferers for many reasons: it's anti-inflammatory, cell protective and vital for collagen synthesis in the skin.[8,9] Collagen is the 'glue' that binds the skin together, making it strong and attractive, and approximately one-third of collagen is composed of glycine. Glycine plays a role in liver detoxification of chemicals and supplementation can significantly reduce salicylate sensitivity.[10] Glycine helps to heal the damaged skin barrier.

Glycine is classed as a 'non-essential' amino acid, as the body is supposed to be able to manufacture its own supply *if your diet is good*. However, in eczema sufferers the ability to manufacturer glycine may not be adequate and/or the glycine receptors in their skin may be compromised. According to researchers from the University of Heidelberg in Germany, people with eczema and psoriasis have a striking reduction in glycine receptors in the skin.[11]

Food sources of glycine

The following is a list of food sources of glycine with the content of glycine listed in milligrams:

- 10g (⅓oz) gelatin, unsweetened dry powder, 1904mg
- broth (Therapeutic Broth, p. 226) (glycine content varies)
- 100g (3½oz) soybeans, raw, 1880mg
- 100g (3½oz) quail, raw, 1542mg
- 100g (3½oz) turkey or chicken with skin, 1395mg
- 100g (3½oz) split peas, raw, 1092mg
- 100g (3½oz) crab meat, blue, 1089mg
- 100g (3½oz) veal, raw, 1078mg
- 100g (3½oz) tuna, raw, 1056mg
- 100g (3½oz) buckwheat, 1031mg
- 100g (3½oz) salmon, raw, 1022mg
- 100g (3½oz) red lentils, raw, 1014mg
- 100g (3½oz) rainbow trout, raw, 1002mg
- 20g (⅔oz) linseeds/flaxseeds, 250mg.

Glycine dosages for eczema sufferers	
Age range	**Glycine total daily intake***
Adults	2000–3000mg (2–3g) (800mg glycine in supplement form)^
13–18 years	800–1000mg (500mg per day in supplement form)^
5–12 years	600–800mg (250–300mg per day in supplement form)^
1–4 years	600mg (125mg per day in supplement form)^
0–12 months	Breastfeeding mothers can take glycine to increase glycine in breastmilk; glycine is in infant formulas but not in adequate amounts. Speak to a nutritionist before giving your baby glycine.

*Total intake from food and supplements.

^Take powdered glycine mixed with water before meals (dosages are in brackets). After your eczema clears up, gradually cut down on the supplement dosage to half the dosage or less. Read 'Dosage note', p. 93.

Tips for breastfeeding mothers

Salicylates end up in breastmilk so babies with eczema and salicylate sensitivity may benefit if their breastfeeding mother takes a glycine, magnesium and vitamin B6 supplement. Also consume Therapeutic Broth (p. 226) daily as it's naturally rich in glycine.

Caution

High-dose glycine taken over long periods of more than six months can cause muscle aches at night, if you are low in oestrogen. If this occurs, discontinue use. Do not take glycine if you are on blood thinning medications such as aspirin, as glycine will reduce the effects of aspirin (it literally detoxifies it). If you are taking medications, seek medical advice before taking liver detoxification supplements.

Powerful co-nutrients

❋ Glycine + magnesium + vitamin B6 (liver detoxification/glycination pathway).

❋ Glycine + cysteine + glutamine (for glutathione) + vitamin B2 + vitamin B6 + vitamin C + brussels sprouts or cabbage (for liver detoxification in the glutathionation pathway).

Biotin

In 1942 a diet experiment was conducted on healthy adults. The volunteers ate white rice, white flour products, sugar, fats, beef and raw egg whites. Within three weeks all the volunteers had itchy, scaly rashes that were diagnosed as eczematous dermatitis. At seven weeks they looked like death with 'striking greyish' skin, indicating poor blood supply to the outer parts of the body.[12,13] Their eczema was not labelled genetic or treated with a topical drug. They were given a biotin supplement and their symptoms completely reversed in less than five days.[14,15]

In 1942, Sydenstricker and colleagues were the first scientists to demonstrate the need for biotin in the diet. They had induced 'egg white injury' where the consumption of avidin, a protein in raw egg whites, latches onto the B-group vitamin called biotin so your body can't use it. Biotin is required for delta-6-desaturase enzyme reactions in the body, and when this enzyme malfunctions from lack of biotin, skin inflammation is the first sign to appear. Biotin deficiency symptoms are: dermatitis or eczema, greyish pallor of the skin, scaly lips, nausea, loss of appetite, depression, moodiness, muscle pain, raised cholesterol and localised numbness.[16,17]

Unfortunately, and despite the research that has been available for more than 60 years, raw egg whites are still present in many supermarket products including dips, whole-egg mayonnaise and coleslaw dressing. Some health experts recommend protein shakes, containing fresh or powdered egg whites. We lick the bowl when making cakes or pancake mix containing raw egg. Traditional chocolate mousse and wedding cake icing contain raw egg whites. It may not be a coincidence that egg allergy is the number one allergy with which eczema sufferers present (and often they're only allergic to raw eggs).[18]

Eating raw egg whites on the rare occasion won't cause problems — egg white injury is achieved if you frequently eat dips, creamy dressings and/or whole-egg mayonnaise and other sources of raw egg whites.

Recommendations

- Check your diet for hidden sources of raw egg whites.
- Tell other people about egg white injury and stop buying products containing raw egg white — food manufacturers will stop using raw egg white in foods such as mayonnaise when consumers stop buying their products.

Food sources of biotin

The following is a list of food sources of biotin with the content of biotin listed in micrograms:

- 100g (3½oz) chicken liver*, 170mcg
- 1 cup cooked soybeans, 40mcg
- 12 oysters, 18mcg
- 1 egg, 15mcg
- 150g (5oz) grilled salmon, 14mcg
- 60g (2⅓oz) rolled (porridge) oats, 12mcg
- 100g (3½oz) canned tuna, 3mcg.

*Liver is the organ that stores and processes chemicals, hormones and pesticides so do not consume liver unless it is organic.

Biotin can be manufactured by friendly bacteria in healthy intestines, yet this may not occur in rash-prone individuals due to genetics, high omega-6 intake, antibiotic use, a bout of diarrhoea or illness. The biotin in food is usually attached to protein and is poorly absorbed by the body, so a biotin supplement is essential for eczema sufferers.

Biotin dosages for eczema sufferers	
Age range	Biotin supplement dosages
Adults	100–150mcg per day in supplement form
5–17 years	50–75mcg per day in supplement form
1–4 years	10–50 mcg per day in supplement form
0–12 months	Obtain biotin through breastmilk if breastfeeding or infant formula or speak to a nutritionist about biotin supplementation.

Caution

High-dose biotin supplementation may lessen the effect of some cholesterol medications.

Powerful co-nutrients

❈ Biotin + vitamin B6 + magnesium + zinc (for delta-6-desaturase enzyme reactions).

Vitamin B6

Vitamin B6 (also known as pyridoxine) is involved in more than 100 enzyme reactions including delta-6-desaturase which helps to reduce inflammation. Vitamin B6 is essential for eczema and allergy sufferers because it's a natural antihistamine and it helps to reduce salicylate and monosodium glutamate (MSG) sensitivity. Vitamin B6 deficiency signs include dermatitis, irritability, mood changes, convulsions, numbness or cramps in the arms and legs, anaemia, smooth painful tongue, ulcers inside the mouth, skin cracks at the corners of the mouth or eyes, low blood sugar/ hypoglycaemia and poor immunity (decreased lymphocytes and interleukin-2).[19,20] Vitamin B6 deficiency can be caused by or is associated with frequent alcohol consumption, poor diet, high-protein diet (this increases the need for vitamin B6), prescription drugs (such as anti-convulsants, anti-turberculosis and penicillamine), cirrhosis of the liver and malabsorption syndromes.

Food sources of vitamin B6

The following is a list of food sources of vitamin B6 with the content of vitamin B6 listed in milligrams:

- 150g (5oz) grilled salmon, 1.2mg
- 60g (2½oz) muesli (granola), 0.96mg
- 40g (1½oz) bran cereal, 0.75mg
- 1 medium potato, 0.7mg
- 2 tablespoons wheatgerm, 0.66mg
- 100g (3½oz) canned tuna, 0.5mg
- 1 cup cooked lentils, 0.45mg
- 150g (5oz) cooked beef, 0.44mg
- 150g (5oz) cooked chicken or turkey, 0.4mg
- 100g (3½oz) brussels sprouts, 0.37mg
- 1 medium banana, 0.35mg
- 80g (3oz) buckwheat, 0.32mg
- 60g (2½oz) rolled (porridge) oats, 0.19mg
- 30g (1oz) cashews, 0.16mg.

Vitamin B6 dosages for eczema sufferers	
Age range	Vitamin B6 supplement dosages
Adults	2mg per day in supplement form
5–17 years	1mg per day in supplement form
1–4 years	0.5–1mg per day in supplement form
0–12 months	0.5mg from breastmilk or infant formula

Caution

If you are taking prescription medications speak to a nutritionist or doctor before taking a vitamin B6 supplement.

Powerful co-nutrients

✳ Vitamin B6 + biotin + magnesium + zinc (anti-inflammatory delta-6-desaturase enzymes).

✳ Vitamin B6 + glycine + magnesium (glycination, Phase 2 liver detoxification).

Magnesium

Magnesium is an alkaline mineral known as 'the great relaxer' as it relieves muscle tension and stiffness, and it can decrease cravings for alcohol. Magnesium is needed for the functioning of more than 300 enzymes in the human body, it helps to alkalise the blood and it decreases chemical sensitivity when combined with glycine and vitamin B6. Magnesium deficiency can be caused by diarrhoea, poor diet, low protein diet (less than 30g/1oz per day), fat malabsorption, frequent alcohol consumption, frequent use of antibiotics or diuretics; and magnesium absorption declines as you age.

Food sources of magnesium

The following is a list of food sources of magnesium with the content of magnesium listed in milligrams:

- 40g (1½oz) processed bran cereal, 115mg
- 60g (2½oz) raw oats, 80mg
- 1 cup cooked brown rice, 80mg
- 1 cup cooked dried beans, 75mg
- 2 tablespoons wheatgerm, 65mg
- 100g (3½oz) prawns, 60mg
- 100g (3½oz) canned sardines, 60mg
- 12 oysters, 60mg
- fish (average serve), 50mg
- chicken or red meat (average serve), 30mg
- 2 slices wholemeal bread, 40mg
- 2 slices white bread, 15mg.

Magnesium dosages for eczema sufferers	
Age range	Magnesium total daily intake* (supplement dosages in brackets)
Adults	350–400mg (200mg in supplement form. The rest should be supplied by a healthy diet.)
5–17 years	240–350mg (100mg per day in supplement form)
1–4 years	130mg (20–50mg per day in supplement form)
0–12 months	30–75mg supplied from breastmilk or infant formula

*Read 'Dosage note', p. 93.

Caution

Magnesium supplementation can interfere with digoxin (heart medicine), some antibiotics, chlorpromazine (tranquiliser), penicillamine, oral anticoagulants and some anti-malaria drugs. Do not take magnesium at the same time as drugs to treat osteoporosis (take them at least 2 hours apart).

Powerful co-nutrients

- ❁ Magnesium + vitamin B6 + biotin + zinc (for delta-6-desaturase enzyme).
- ❁ Magnesium + vitamin B6 + glycine (glycination, Phase 2 liver detoxification).

Zinc

Zinc is vital for skin repair and maintenance and deficiency leads to skin lesions, dry and rough skin and delayed wound healing. A severe zinc deficiency, caused by faulty gene expression, induces bullous pustular dermatitis (blister-like dermatitis), patches of eczema and hair loss (alopecia).[21] Other deficiency signs include acne, stretch marks, white-coated tongue, white spots on fingernails, impotence, infertility, frequent infections, frizzy hair, poor sense of taste or smell and premature ageing of the skin. During your teenage years, rapid development requires zinc and these growth spurts can lead to zinc deficiency, and as the skin's oil gland activity is regulated by zinc, acne can result.

Menstruation and ejaculation deplete zinc stores in the body and zinc deficiency can be caused by frequent alcohol consumption, high salt intake (from canned food, takeaway/restaurant food), high calcium intake, chronic stress, frequent consumption of coffee or tea, and high fibre diets rich in phytic acid (which is why soaking grains is recommended, see p. 80).

Food sources of zinc

The following is a list of food sources of zinc with the content of zinc listed in milligrams:

- 12 oysters, approx. 54–76mg
- 150g (5oz) cooked lamb shank, 14.5mg
- 100g (3½oz) cooked crab, 9.1mg
- 150g (5oz) cooked beef, 7.7mg
- 150g (5oz) cooked lamb, 6.4mg
- 100g (3½oz) dried beans, 3mg
- 100g (3½oz) raw brown rice, 2.1mg
- 60g (2½oz) muesli (granola), 1.8mg
- 100g (3½oz) cooked prawns, 1.8mg
- 100g (3½oz) peas, 1.8mg
- 2 tablespoons wheatgerm, 1.5mg
- 60g (2½oz) rolled (porridge) oats, 1.1mg
- 100g (3½oz) raw white rice, 1.1mg
- 2 slices wholemeal bread, 0.9mg
- 2 slices white bread, 0.4mg.

Testing for zinc deficiency

You can do a simple zinc taste test to confirm if you have a zinc deficiency. This test is often available from health food shops, naturopaths and naturopathic clinics. When you have a measured dose of liquid zinc, hold it in your mouth for a few seconds before swallowing it or spitting it out. Your tastebuds will indicate the degree of need for zinc supplementation: if you have a deficiency, the mixture will taste like water, be pleasant tasting or leave a furry feeling in the mouth. If your body has plenty of stored zinc, the liquid will taste metallic or foul and you'll probably want to spit it out.

Zinc dosages for eczema sufferers	
Age range	Zinc daily intake
Adults	8mg in supplement form*
5–17 years	4mg in supplement form*
1–4 years	2mg supplement*
0–12 months	2–4mg supplied from breastmilk or infant formula

*Salt and supplements containing calcium, iron and/or phosphorus can prevent zinc supplements from being absorbed so, if possible, have your zinc supplement 1 to 2 hours apart from these substances.

Caution

Do not take zinc supplements if you have copper deficiency or if you're taking tetracycline (a drug for infections) as zinc competes for absorption with copper and may make your medical treatment less effective. Do not exceed the prescribed dosage as excessive zinc intake can cause diarrhoea, abdominal pains, nausea, dehydration, dizziness and lethargy.

Powerful co-nutrients

- ❀ Zinc + magnesium + vitamin B6 + biotin (for delta-6-desaturase enzyme).
- ❀ Zinc + magnesium + B-group vitamins (to detoxify amines, hormones and alcohol in Phase 2 liver detoxification).

Chromium

The mineral chromium is required in micro amounts for normal growth and general health. In 1959 it was identified as the active ingredient in 'glucose tolerance factor' and it enhances the action of the hormone insulin, which helps your body process glucose in the blood. Chromium is needed for the breakdown of proteins, carbohydrates and fats and it enhances the body's ability to convert glucose to energy. It is not a miracle nutrient or a 'wonder' supplement but for those who are deficient in chromium, supplementation can greatly improve their energy levels, ability to think clearly and quality of life.

In the 1800s carbohydrate avoidance was recommended as part of a diet that prevented eczema; however, with additional information about the benefits of chromium supplementation, total carbohydrate avoidance is not necessary or advised (as you need dietary fibre for gastrointestinal health). Chromium supplementation enables sufferers to be able to enjoy good quality wholegrain carbohydrates while on the Eczema Diet.

Food sources of chromium

The following is a list of food sources of chromium with the content of chromium listed in micrograms:

- 2 cups cos (romaine) lettuce, 15.6mcg
- ½ cup raw onion, 12.4mcg
- 100g (3½oz) turkey meat, 10.4mcg
- 1 cup cooked peas, 6mcg
- 1 teaspoon dried garlic, 3mcg
- 1 cup mashed potato, 3mcg
- 2 slices wholemeal bread, 2mcg
- 1 medium banana, 1mcg
- ½ cup green beans, 1mcg.

Modern Western diets are low in chromium and generally rich in processed carbohydrates and frequent sugar consumption is considered normal, causing an increased need for chromium in the diet. Chromium supplementation can decrease sugar cravings and cravings for carbohydrates and it can reduce excessive hunger, fatigue (especially after meals or afternoon energy slumps), glucose intolerance and irritability (adding cinnamon to the diet can also lower blood glucose and increase insulin sensitivity — however, cinnamon is high in salicylates and only suitable in Stage 2 of the Eczema Diet).

Chromium dosages for eczema sufferers	
Age range	Chromium daily intake
Adults	90mcg in supplement form
5–17 years	45mcg in supplement form
1–4 years	13–25mcg
0–12 months	1–7mcg from breastmilk or infant formula

Adequate intake (AI) of 25mcg elemental chromium is equivalent to 200mcg of chromium picolinate.

While statistics on chromium deficiency are limited, data from research suggests that only 0.4–2.5 per cent of chromium is absorbed from foods. Vitamin C and vitamin B3 (niacin) enhance the absorption of chromium, as does protein, so take a chromium supplement with a protein-rich meal.[22] Chromium picolinate is easier for the body to absorb than other types of chromium and a chromium supplement should also contain B6, B12, vitamin C, vitamin D3, folic acid, magnesium and zinc.

Caution

If you are taking medical drugs, consult with a nutritionist or doctor before taking chromium. If you have insulin-dependent diabetes seek advice from your doctor before supplementing with chromium as it alters blood sugar levels (insulin would need to be reduced if you were taking chromium but do this only with your doctor's supervision).

Powerful co-nutrients

❋ Chromium + vitamin C + vitamin B3 + protein (to enhance absorption).

Vitamin D

Vitamin D is manufactured in the skin after direct sunlight exposure and it's obtained through your diet. It's an important fat-soluble vitamin that directly and indirectly controls more than 200 genes (so if vitamin D is deficient how does this affect your genetics?). According to Sidbury and colleagues from the Children's Hospital in Boston, children with moderate to severe atopic eczema have significantly lower levels of vitamin D compared with children who have mild symptoms.[23] A study by the same researchers found that adults with eczema consume diets lower in vitamin D than people without eczema.

Vitamin D deficiency is common, especially in cooler climates, and more than 1 billion people worldwide have vitamin D deficiency or insufficiency.[24] Deficiency is linked to a range of health problems including rickets, poor bone health, severe fatigue, psoriasis, muscle weakness and a 30 to 50 per cent increased risk of cancers of the colon, prostate and breast.[25,26,27]

What can diminish vitamin D in the body? Low or inadequate exposure to direct sunlight is the main contributing factor. This can occur in winter or cooler climates and from overuse of protective clothing and sunscreens. According to research published in the *British Journal of Dermatology*, frequent use of cortisone cream depletes vitamin D in the skin.[28] When you use topical steroids or other topical drugs prescribed for eczema you are advised to avoid direct sun exposure as topical steroids make the skin fragile and more prone to sun damage. Which highlights another reason why we need to adopt healthy alternatives to medicated creams.

Frequent, small exposures to sunlight help to restore vitamin D levels as does a healthy diet and supplementation, which is highly recommended for eczema sufferers.

Food sources of vitamin D

The following is a list of food sources of vitamin D with the content of vitamin D listed in micrograms:

- 100g (3½oz) grilled herring, 25mcg
- 100g (3½oz) canned red salmon, 23.1mcg
- 100g (3½oz) canned pink salmon, 17mcg
- 150g (5oz) grilled trout, 16.5mcg

- 150g (5oz) grilled salmon, 14.4mcg
- 150g (5oz) tuna, fresh, 10.8mcg
- 100g (3½oz) cooked kippers, 9.4mcg
- 100g (3½oz) cooked mackerel, 5.4mcg
- 100g (3½oz) canned tuna in brine, 3mcg.

Recommendations

- Ask your doctor to check your vitamin D level.
- Make sure adequate amounts of vitamin D are being consumed in your diet.
- Have safe sun exposure daily: about 10 minutes every day of unfiltered sunshine directly on the skin will keep vitamin D deficiency away in healthy individuals. If you have eczema and/or vitamin D deficiency a supplement is advised.

Vitamin D dosages for eczema sufferers	
Age range	Vitamin D3 daily intake
Adults	400–800 IU in supplement form
5–17 years	200–400 IU in supplement form
1–4 years	100–200 IU in supplement form
0–12 months	5–15mcg from breastmilk or infant formula

1mcg of vitamin D = 40 IU (international units).

Caution

If you have diabetes speak to your doctor before taking vitamin D as it may lower blood sugar levels. You may not be able to take vitamin D if you have kidney disease, kidney stones or granulomatous disease (immune disorder), as increased vitamin D intake may increase calcium in the blood.

Powerful co-nutrients

❋ Vitamin D + calcium + magnesium + vitamin K (for bone health).

Vitamin E

Vitamin E is the predominant antioxidant in human skin.[29] Supplementation can decrease the allergy marker immunoglobulin E (IgE) in allergy sufferers, improve immune responses and decrease the production and release of pro-inflammatory prostaglandins. A clinical trial published in the *International Journal of Dermatology* revealed that nearly 50 per cent of adults with atopic dermatitis who were treated with 400 IU (268mg) of vitamin E daily for eight months showed great improvement (compared to only one in the placebo group); and there was almost complete remission of atopic eczema in seven people taking the vitamin E, but none in the placebo group (four of the adults treated with vitamin E worsened, compared to 36 in the placebo).[30] While this study showed promising results, other studies have not been so positive and it must be stressed that vitamin E should be taken with vitamin C and alpha-lipoic acid so you don't need to take the mega dose of vitamin E used in this study (vitamin C and alpha-lipoic acid recycle vitamin E, helping it to circulate for longer).

Food sources of vitamin E

The following is a list of food sources of vitamin E with the content of vitamin E listed in milligrams:

- 20ml (½fl oz) sunflower oil, 9.8mg
- 100g (3½oz) cabbage, 0.2–7mg*
- 100g (3½oz) sweet potato, 4.6mg
- 150g (5oz) grilled salmon, 3.5mg
- 100g (3½oz) prawns, 2.9mg
- 1 cup cooked soybeans, 2.2mg
- 1 cup cooked chickpeas (garbanzo beans), 2mg
- 100g (3½oz) canned red salmon, 2.1mg
- 100g (3½oz) canned tuna in oil, 1.9mg
- 100g (3½oz) canned pink salmon, 1.5mg
- 100g (3½oz) brussels sprouts, 1mg
- 100g (3½oz) leeks, 0.9mg
- 100g (3½oz) lettuce, 0.6mg
- ½ cup raw carrots, 0.4mg
  (*Green outer leaves of cabbage contain 7mg vitamin E; the white inner leaves have only 0.2mg.)

Vitamin E dosages for eczema sufferers	
Age range	Vitamin E daily intake
Adults	40mg in supplement form
5–17 years	20mg in supplement form
1–4 years	10mg in supplement form
0–12 months	4–5mg (6–7.5 IU) (AI) from breastmilk or infant formula

Take vitamin E (d-alpha-tocopherol) with vitamin C and alpha-lipoic acid.

1 IU (international unit) of vitamin E is equivalent to 0.67mg of vitamin E. To convert IUs into mg (milligrams): multiply the number of IUs by 0.67.

Vitamin E from natural food sources is called 'd-alpha-tocopherol' and it's more potent than the synthetic form. Synthetic vitamin E is listed as 'dl-alpha-tocopherol' and this artificial form (denoted by 'dl') should not be taken.

Caution

Vitamin E thins the blood so do not take vitamin E if you are on blood-thinning medications such as aspirin or if you are undergoing surgery. If you are on any medications, consult with your doctor before taking vitamin E.

Powerful co-nutrients

- ❋ Vitamin E + vitamin C + alpha-lipoic acid (antioxidant protection).
- ❋ Vitamin E + quercetin (blocks pro-inflammatory leukotriene formation).

Quercetin

Quercetin is a potent antioxidant flavonoid found in fruits and vegetables and it's the major therapeutic ingredient in onions and various herbal medicines. Quercetin is a natural antihistamine as it reduces blood histamine levels and it can help to reverse the liver damage caused by nitrate consumption.[31,32] When combined with vitamin C it can quickly reduce and prevent hay fever symptoms. Quercetin is anti-inflammatory as it inhibits the formation of pro-inflammatory leukotrienes, which are associated with eczema and asthma (see Diagram 3, 'How prostaglandins control inflammation', p. 30). Quercetin can be taken in supplement form, but it is best consumed in your diet. *The Eczema Diet* recipes are rich in quercetin.

Food sources of quercetin

The following is a list of food sources of quercetin with the content of quercetin listed in milligrams:

- 100g (3½oz) buckwheat, 15–36mg
- 50g (2oz) elderberries*, raw, 21mg
- 50g (2oz) onions*, cooked, 9.9mg
- 100g (3½oz) buckwheat flour, 2.7mg
- 100g (3½oz) buckwheat groats, roasted, 2–8.7mg
- 100g (3½oz) blueberries*, raw or frozen, 2–7.3mg
- 50g (2oz) raw spring onions (scallions), 7.1mg
- 100g (3½oz) apple*, with skin, 4.4mg
- 100g (3½oz) yellow beans, snap, raw, 3mg
- 100g (3½oz) celery, raw, 3.5mg
- 100g (3½oz) apple*, skinless, 1.5mg
- 100g (3½oz) green beans, raw, 2.7mg
- 100g (3½oz) iceberg lettuce, 2.4mg
- 50g (2oz) cherries*, canned, 1.6mg
- 50g (2oz) bilberries*, raw, 1.5mg
- 100g (3½oz) green beans, frozen, cooked, 1.2mg
- 100g (3½oz) pear, raw, 0.4mg.

*This food may not be eczema-safe.

Essential fatty acids

Essential fatty acids (EFAs) are vital for healthy skin and are classified as 'essential' fats because your body cannot manufacture them and they must be obtained from your diet. The two main groups of essential fatty acids are omega-3 and omega-6. Rich sources of omega-3 include linseeds/flaxseeds and fish, especially trout, salmon and sardines (eczema-safe fish are listed on p. 72).

To demonstrate how diet influences the skin, scientists De Spirt and colleagues gave two groups of women either flaxseed or borage oil for twelve weeks and a third group received a placebo which was olive oil. After six weeks of consuming ½ teaspoon of either flaxseed oil or borage oil, skin water loss was decreased by about 10 per cent, and by week twelve the flaxseed oil group showed further protection from water loss and the skin was significantly more hydrated. While the olive oil (placebo) group had no significant change, at twelve weeks the flaxseed-oil group had significantly less skin reddening (after irritation), roughness and scaling of the skin.[33]

Do all fats increase skin moisture content?

No. Olive oil contains mostly omega-9 which does not influence skin hydration, and saturated fats, from meat and dairy products, promote dry skin in eczema sufferers. Research shows that diets high in fats, where 10 per cent of energy is consumed as saturated fat and monounsaturated fat (from vegetable oils, margarine and nuts), decreases skin hydration and increases the skin's surface pH, *making the skin more susceptible to microbe invasion and bacterial infections.*[34]

For flaxseed oil dosages refer to p. 70.

Omega-3 diet recommendations

Eczema sufferers may not digest or utilise fats adequately due to genetics or faulty enzyme conversions. I recommend eczema sufferers obtain their omega-3 from food sources rather than taking a supplement as the oil is better absorbed from foods. If you experience beneficial effects from taking fish oil supplements, and you would like to take them, look for supplements that are unflavoured and colour-free (children's fish oil supplements usually contain natural or artificial flavours so they are not eczema-safe).

Eat eczema-safe fish twice a week (read 'Safe seafood', p. 72). Have whole or ground linseeds/flaxseeds or fresh flaxseed oil daily. Flaxseed oil and oil supplements should be taken with soy lecithin granules to increase absorption (lecithin information is on p. 74). Recipes include Healthy Skin Smoothie, p. 223; and in Stage 2 only, Flaxseed Lemon Drink, p. 223.

Food sources of omega-3

The following is a list of food sources of omega-3 with the content of omega-3 listed in milligrams:

- 113g (4oz) salmon, 2000mg
- 1 tablespoon linseeds/flaxseeds, 1750mg
- 2 x omega-3 fortified eggs, 1114mg
- 113g (4oz) scallops, 1100mg
- 1 cup soybeans, 700mg
- 113g (4oz) halibut, baked, 620mg
- 113g (4oz) tofu, 360mg
- 1 cup baby (pattypan) squash, 340mg
- 1 cup cabbage, 170mg

Food sources of EPA and DHA

EPA (eicosapentaenoic acid) and DHA (docosahexaenoic acid) are omega-3 in its converted and more potent form. Many of the health benefits of omega-3 are attributed to EPA and DHA. EPA/DHA are also present in the foods listed below, especially coldwater fish:

- 100g (3½oz) Atlantic salmon, 1090–1830mg*
- 100g (3½oz) fresh tuna, 240–1280mg*
- 100g (3½oz) herring, 1710–1810mg*
- 100g (3½oz) sardines, 980–1700mg*
- 100g (3½oz) rainbow trout, 840–980mg*
- 100g (3½oz) mackerel, 340–1570mg*
- 100g (3½oz) canned tuna in water, drained, 260–730mg*
- 1 tablespoon flaxseed oil, 850mg
- 1 tablespoon linseeds, ground or whole, 220mg
- 2 slices soy linseed bread, 180mg

*The EPA and DHA content varies depending on whether the skin has been left on or removed: fish with the skin on are higher in fat so they are richer sources of omega-3 fatty acids, EPA and DHA.

Caution

Acne: Do not take flaxseed oil, omega-3 oils, evening primrose oil or any oil supplement if you have acne, as doing so may increase skin oiliness.

If you choose to take an omega-3 fish oil supplement be aware that it thins the blood and this increases the risk of bleeding, so discontinue use several weeks before surgery or childbirth. Do not take oil supplements if you are on blood-thinning (heart) medications such as aspirin and seek advice from a nutritionist if you are on any medications.

Probiotics

Probiotics contain health-promoting bacteria, also known as microflora, which are naturally found in the gastrointestinal tract of healthy people. At birth an infant's gastrointestinal tract contains no bacteria — it is sterile — then during the first year of life colonisation begins and (ideally) a healthy range of bacteria is established. Microflora work by adhering to your gut wall and 'policing' potentially harmful microbes so they can't multiply and thrive. Beneficial bacteria promote healthy digestion and they can manufacture some vitamins, including the B-group vitamins, so they help to decrease the risk of nutritional deficiencies.

Unfortunately, beneficial microflora are not always present in adequate amounts. Microflora imbalance or deficiency is associated with antibiotic use, illness, diarrhoea and/or poor health of the gastrointestinal tract. Microflora imbalance allows pathogens, such as *Candida albicans*, to thrive in the gastrointestinal tract and this increases the risk of food intolerances and itchy skin. Research shows that an altered ratio of the microflora strains can precede the development of atopic eczema.[35] According to one such study, the presence of the bacterial strains *Escherichia coli* and *Clostridium difficile* is associated with an increased risk of eczema and allergies at two years of age.[36] The research suggests that probiotics can promote proper gut barrier function and healing of intestinal permeability. In some (but not all) studies, probiotics decreased allergic inflammation in eczema sufferers.

Microflora imbalances

The signs that indicate you may have a microflora imbalance or deficiency include:

- skin inflammation
- itchy skin
- *Candida albicans* infestation (symptoms are listed on p. 24 in the candida questionnaire)
- allergies and increased sensitivities
- cravings for sugar
- white fungal patches on the skin
- biotin deficiency (and other B-group vitamins)
- gastrointestinal dysfunction (diarrhoea or constipation, foul smelling gas and/or stools, bloating, abdominal pain, poor digestion).

These symptoms can also be caused by other conditions and should be discussed with your doctor. Microflora imbalance can be caused by or is associated with the following factors:

- Caesarean or premature birth
- if the mother had a candida infection in the vaginal tract at the time of giving birth
- use of oral antibiotics
- illness
- diarrhoea
- compromised gut function
- gut lining permeability
- high-sugar diets (acid-promoting diets)
- immune system dysfunction
- use of the birth control pill
- hormone replacement therapy
- corticosteroids (e.g. hydrocortisone)
- excessive consumption of processed foods including refined carbohydrates (white bread, cake, biscuits, soft drink/sodas), sugar (including in soft drinks, cordial, fruit juice)
- frequent consumption of alcohol.

Different types of microflora — which ones are best for eczema?

The beneficial bacteria in probiotics come from two groups: Lactobacillus and Bifidobacterium. Within these groups are different strains such as *Lactobacillus acidophilus* and *Bifidobacterium animalis*. Please keep in mind that the benefits from probiotics are strain-specific. For example the strain *L. acidophilus* LA5 does not treat eczema (it helps conditions such as *Candida albicans*) but the strain known as *L. rhamnosus* GG was found to improve eczema symptoms in 50 per cent of children with eczema.[37] Probiotics should be used after an eczema sufferer has taken a course of antibiotics, been ill, had diarrhoea, experienced an adverse or allergic reaction to food, or if you have compromised gut function, dandruff, *Candida albicans* or fungal infestation. When choosing a probiotic supplement look at the ingredients panel for the specific strain of probiotic (e.g. *L. rhamnosus* GG). Probiotics are generally safe for infants and you can speak to a doctor or nutritionist regarding probiotics for your child.

Condition	Suitable probiotic strains [38-45]
eczema	*Lactobacillus rhamnosus* GG (also known as LGG or *Lactobacillus* GG) *Lactobacillus* F79 *Bifidobacterium animalis*, (also called *B. animalis* or *B. lactis* Bb12 or *Bifidobacterium lactis* Bb12) *Lactobacillus fermentum* PCC *Lactobacillus reuteri* ATCC 55730 (*L. reuteri*) *L. reuteri* DSM 122460 (combined with *L. rhamnosus* GG)
Candida albicans	*Lactobacillus acidophilus* LA5 *Lactobacillus rhamnosus* GG *Lactobacillus acidophilus* strain NAS *Lactobacillus acidophilus* NCFM
digestive dysfunction	*Lactobacillus rhamnosus* GG *Bifidobacterium animalis* *Lactobacillus johnsonii* La1 *Lactobacillus plantarum* 299v *Lactobacillus paracasei* Shirota *Propionibacterium freudenreichii* HA-101 and HA-102 sauerkraut (probiotic food)

Condition	Suitable probiotic strains [38-45]
allergies	Lactobacillus rhamnosus GG
	Lactobacillus johnsonii La1
antibiotic use	Lactobacillus rhamnosus GG (L. rhamnosus GG)
	Lactobacillus acidophilus LA5

Probiotic dosages for eczema sufferers	
Age range	**Probiotic daily intake**
Children and adults	Refer to product label or speak to a nutritionist for dosage.*
0–12 months	Refer to product label or speak to a nutritionist for dosage. Breastfeeding mothers: take the supplement yourself and put a few grains of probiotic onto your nipple before breastfeeding (do this twice daily); a tiny sprinkling of suitable probiotics can be added to lukewarm infant formula or sprinkled onto baby rice cereal twice daily.

*Have a suitable probiotic supplement twice a day, mixed in a little water or rice milk, taken before breakfast and in the afternoon. If serving probiotics to small children you can also sprinkle probiotic grains onto cold cereal or cooled baby rice cereal (don't add probiotics to overly warm foods) or add it to their milk bottle after the milk has been warmed.

Caution

Discontinue use of probiotics if diarrhoea or constipation occurs.

Carotenoids

Research shows that eating foods rich in cryptoxanthin, a carotenoid that supplies vitamin A, can help to *increase* skin hydration when consumed as part of a healthy diet.[46] Fat-soluble vitamin A has the opposite effect — it dries out the skin — and should not be taken in supplement form unless vitamin A deficiency has been diagnosed. Cryptoxanthin-rich foods include papaya and pawpaw, which can be consumed daily (they're also rich in vitamin C). Other carotenoid-rich foods that are eczema-safe and vital for eczema sufferers include carrots, beetroot and sweet potato. Have at least one carotenoid-rich fruit or vegetable daily.

Calcium

Calcium is the most abundant mineral in the body and it's stored in your bones. The body regulates a constant level of calcium in the blood in order to keep the blood pH slightly alkaline, and this is beneficial for bone and skin health. In a study by Boelsma and colleagues, calcium helped to improve the acid mantle of the skin,[47] so calcium may increase the skin's ability to protect itself against dust mite invasion and infections. The epidermis layer of the skin must also respond to weather extremes and calcium helps to maintain the right amount of moisturising lipids by triggering their production in low humidity or when required. These lipids are water-resistant so they trap water in the skin so it does not dry out. The calcium paradox is that dairy products can contribute to eczema, while calcium *in supplement form* is beneficial for eczema as it boosts moisture levels in the skin, decreases the itch and promotes a more restful night's sleep.

Food sources of calcium

The following is a list of eczema-safe food sources of calcium with the content of calcium listed in milligrams:

- 1 cup calcium-fortified soy milk or rice milk, 300mg
- 100g (3½oz) canned or fresh sardines, 300mg
- 100g (3½oz) canned or fresh salmon, 200–300mg
- ½ cup cooked green soybeans, 130mg
- 1 bowl oatmeal/porridge, 99–110mg
- ½ cup canned or fresh white beans, 96mg
- 160g (5⅓oz) fish fillet, 85mg
- 80g (3oz) cooked rainbow trout, 73mg
- 100g (3½oz) cabbage, 40mg

Calcium dosages for eczema sufferers	
Age range	Calcium daily intake from supplement sources
Adults	800mg
During pregnancy, breastfeeding and lactation, and menopause	1200mg

Calcium dosages for eczema sufferers	
Age range	Calcium daily intake from supplement sources
5–17 years	400mg
1–4 years	400mg
Infants 7–12 months old	270mg from breastmilk or infant formula, and food if on solids
Infants 0–6 months old	210mg from breastmilk or infant formula

It is essential to take a calcium supplement while on the Eczema Diet, and powder or chewable gummy supplements are available if you cannot swallow large tablets (avoid artificially sweetened products). Calcium is best taken in calcium citrate form. Take calcium citrate combined with calcium carbonate, magnesium and vitamin D to promote absorption, and ideally have it on an empty stomach in the afternoon and/or before bed.

Caution

Combined dietary and supplemental intake of calcium should not exceed 2500mg per day as excessive calcium can cause adverse reactions. Do not take calcium if you have kidney failure, kidney stones, hyperparathyroidism, sarcoidosis or cancer. Calcium supplementation can interfere with medications so speak to your doctor if you take medications. Do not take antacids containing aluminium as calcium can significantly increase the amount of aluminium absorbed into the blood.[48] (If you need antacids it's a sign your diet is too high in acid. See acid–alkaline balance information on p. 50.)

Supplements to avoid or limit

The following is a list of supplements best avoided by those with eczema.

Supplements containing herbs

Some herbal medicines can be beneficial for rashes but they may also cause adverse effects, especially if you have salicylate sensitivity, so they should only be taken if prescribed by a naturopath or herbalist. All herbal medicines, including St Mary's Thistle which is in most liver detoxification supplements, are rich in natural plant chemicals such as salicylates. Green tea (in both tea form and in supplements) and supplement ingredients such as 'vegetable extracts', broccoli, wheatgrass juice and barley grass all contain very high levels of salicylates so they are not eczema-safe. However, herbal medicines prescribed for treating *Candida albicans* infestations can be beneficial to take before or during the Eczema Diet if a fungal infection has been diagnosed.

Vitamin A

Fat-soluble vitamin A (retinol) helps to mop up excess oil in the skin so it decreases skin moisture, which is beneficial if you have acne but not good for eczema and dry skin. High intake of vitamin A is associated with a significant increase in surface pH (in women) and again this is not good for eczema sufferers who need a lower, acidic pH to guard against invading bacteria.[49] For this reason, eczema sufferers should not take a supplement containing vitamin A or cod liver oil or eat liver (e.g. lamb's fry) without first consulting a nutritionist.

Keep in mind that you need vitamin A in your diet to avoid deficiency and you will obtain a safe amount of vitamin A from red meat, chicken, seafood and orange-coloured vegetables such as carrot and sweet potato (in the form of beta-carotene). Babies do not adequately convert beta-carotene into retinol so, to avoid deficiency, infants need dietary retinol/vitamin A from breastmilk, infant formula and/or finely ground meats when on solids.[50]

Key points to remember

This chapter covered a wide range of supplements and not all of them are absolutely essential to take during the program (for example, fish oil supplements). So to avoid confusion, here are the main supplements recommended during the Eczema Diet:

1. Take a daily supplement containing vitamin C, glycine, vitamin B6, magnesium, natural vitamin E, biotin, zinc and chromium. Once your eczema improves, reduce the dosages.

2. Consume whole or ground linseeds/flaxseeds daily (see p. 70) or add flaxseed oil to the Healthy Skin Smoothie, p. 223.

3. Take a *dairy-free* probiotic supplement for eczema, for one to two courses (1–2 bottles) or after taking antibiotics, and after suffering from diarrhoea or fungal infestation (see 'Probiotics', p. 113).

4. Take a calcium citrate supplement, with added magnesium and vitamin D, on an empty stomach in between meals. Take calcium on an ongoing basis.

Note: Over the years I've had many people contact me regarding supplements for eczema, as they can be very difficult to find, so I am bringing out an eczema supplement range to make this program easier to follow. See www.beautyby.com.au for product information.

Part 2

Non-diet information

On the first day, the head was painted with a 'lotion' of durrameal and fruit-of-the-dompalm, warmed in soft fat and was bound up. On the second day, the head was anointed with fish oil; on the fourth day with abra oil. After this course of intensive treatment the offending head, if the eczema still persisted, was smeared daily with breadmeal and dressed with rotted cereals.

—The first recorded treatment for eczema, from ancient Egypt (Wright, 1979)

Chapter 7
Skin care products, make-up + daily regime

Your skin is constructed, repaired and maintained using nutrients obtained from your daily diet. However, when you have eczema a little extra help from the outside is a welcome relief too. A healthy skin care routine can speed up the healing process and soothe the itch. On the other hand, the wrong skin care routine can damage the skin barrier function and delay healing, so let's begin by looking at the skin care ingredients to avoid.

Problematic ingredient	Uses (found in)	Problems
Sulfates: especially sodium lauryl sulfate (SLS) Milder sulfates include: sodium lauryth sulfate, sodium C14–16 olefin sulfate, TEA-lauryl sulfate	Foaming detergent, emulsifier (foaming toiletries, aqueous cream, commercial toothpastes, shampoos, cleansers, hand wash, baby shampoos and bubble bath)	SLS can cause contact dermatitis, alters the skin's pH, thins the skin barrier (damage can last for 4 weeks after use), water loss from the skin, rashes, dandruff, hair loss and dry skin (Tip: favour 'sulfate-free' products)
Formaldehyde (formaldehyde and its derivatives imidazolidinyl urea and DMDM hydantoin)	Preservative (shampoos, liquid hand soap, hair products, hair gel, cosmetics, nail polish and moisturisers)	Releases formaldehyde, skin irritant, allergic reactions/rashes and it may affect breathing in asthmatics
Fragrance (4000 varieties of fragrance or 'parfum', many are synthetic)	Hides undesirable smells (moisturisers, cosmetics, deodorant, cleansers, hair conditioners and shampoos, baby shampoo, perfumes, cosmetics and colognes)	Aggravates hand eczema, dermatitis, dizziness, hyperpigmentation of the skin, hyperactivity and irritation in children and some adults (Tip: choose products labelled 'fragrance-free')

Problematic ingredient	Uses (found in)	Problems
Isopropyl alcohol (isopropanol)	Anti-bacterial solvent made from petroleum (toners, shaving creams and other men's skin care products)	Drying and irritating, strips the skin's natural acid mantle making it vulnerable to bacteria and fungus, promotes liver spots and pigmentation, and can irritate the eyes and skin
DEA and MEA (such as lauramide DEA, cocamide DEA, and cocamide MEA)	Emulsifier used to mix oil and water in products and a foaming agent (shampoos)	Contact allergies such as skin rashes

Skin care ingredients to favour

There is not one definitive group of skin care ingredients that will be eczema-safe for everyone. For example, I've had eczema patients who say plain sorbolene cream is the only product their skin can tolerate, while others find sorbolene cream irritates their skin and yet natural, herbal-based moisturisers offer them some relief. So this list has been compiled with a lot of thought and comes with a note of caution: as your skin is broken, irritation can occur, so always test a product on undamaged skin before applying to your eczema.

The following ingredients work best when used *within* a skin care product containing a range of ingredients, and it is not necessary or advised to use all these ingredients at once.

Beneficial skin care ingredients	Properties
Aloe vera	Anti-inflammatory, anti-bacterial
Blackcurrant seed oil (*Ribes nigrum*)	Anti-inflammatory, moisturising properties, omega-3
Borage oil	Anti-inflammatory, contains gamma-linolenic acid (GLA) and omega-3
Calendula (*Calendula officinalis*)	Anti-inflammatory, antiseptic, anti-bacterial and astringent, flavonoids

Beneficial skin care ingredients	Properties
Chamomile (Anthemis nobilis)	Astringent, anti-bacterial, anti-inflammatory, contains fatty acids, rutin and quercetin
Cocoa butter	Moisturising properties, contains antioxidants such as vitamin E
Emu oil	Anti-inflammatory, essential fatty acids, omega-3
Evening primrose oil	Anti-inflammatory, contains gamma-linolenic acid (GLA)
Jojoba oil	Protects skin from water loss, similar to your skin's own sebum
Licorice root/licorice extract (Glycyrrhiza glabra)	Anti-inflammatory, anti-viral, anti-bacterial
Manuka honey	Anti-inflammatory, anti-bacterial, antioxidants, moisturising
Rosehip oil (good quality rosehip oil should be a rich amber colour)	Moisturising properties, antioxidants, vitamin C, transretinoic acid (natural vitamin A), lycopene, carotenoids, essential fatty acids
Sea buckthorn berry oil	Anti-inflammatory, moisturising properties, antioxidants (vitamins A, C and E), unique 1:1 ratio of omega-3 and omega-6 oils, palmitoleic acid (a fatty acid in human skin sebum)
Shea butter (Butyrospermum parkii)	Excellent moisturising properties, contains fatty acids and a small amount of natural UV factor, anti-inflammatory
Vitamin E, natural (d-alpha-tocopherol or tocopherol)	Natural preservative and antioxidant (do not use oils that are 100 per cent vitamin E oil as they may cause pigmentation of the skin and avoid synthetic 'dl' vitamin E such as 'dl-alpha-tocopherol')

Essential oils

Natural essential oils blended into an eczema cream may be beneficial for the skin, however keep in mind they can also cause skin irritation, especially if you are sensitive to salicylates.

Preservatives

Unpreserved or poorly preserved skin care products can become contaminated with bacteria and can lead to bacterial infections if you have broken skin such as eczema. To reduce the risk of contaminating your skin care products, do not put your fingers into pots of ointment or skin creams, and throw out older products. Although there is a risk of stinging from preserved skin care products, favour products that are preserved.

Skin care products

Various types of moisturisers are collectively referred to as 'emollients'. The following list of emollients, listed from thickest to thinnest in consistency, can help to make shopping for a skin care product easier.

Ointments

Ointments, such as Vaseline and pawpaw ointment, are thick and greasy and they are useful for scaly skin and extremely dry patches. A thick coat of ointment can protect your skin from stinging when you go for a swim in the ocean or chlorinated pool (although it's best to avoid chlorine if you can help it). On the down side, ointments can stain your clothes and they can cause rebound dryness when you stop using the product. Vaseline and pawpaw ointments are petroleum-based, however there are petroleum-free pawpaw ointments available. According to the National Eczema Society in the United Kingdom, ointments do not contain preservatives so they should not be used on weeping eczema or broken skin.

Note: It is important to avoid putting your fingers into the pot of ointment as bacterial contamination can occur. Use a clean utensil to transfer some of the ointment into another clean container before applying.

Moisturisers

Studies show that damaged skin barrier function can be partially restored by applying oil-based moisturisers as they contain fatty acids and other nutrients and help to prevent water loss. On the down side, moisturisers may not be protective enough for very dry and irritated skin. When eczema flares up, a non-irritating moisturiser can be applied two to four times daily, and in severe cases up to six times a day.

Creams and lotions

These are thin in consistency and rapidly soak into the skin. On the down side, creams and lotions need to be reapplied more often and they may not offer enough protection for very dry and itchy skin.

Note: Before purchasing an emollient check the ingredient list and, if possible, test it on a patch of healthy, unbroken skin to see if irritation occurs.

Hand washes and soaps

Normal, healthy skin should have a pH of 5.5 but after soap use the skin's pH increases to more than 7.5. This is because most soaps and cleansing products are highly alkaline (with a pH range of 9–11). Most cleansing products also contain sulfates so they disrupt the skin's protective acid mantle and break down the skin's valuable barrier. Skin cleansers, soaps, detergents and other foaming agents can cause dryness, swelling, flaking, tightness, roughness and thinning of the skin barrier and they can leave the skin vulnerable to microbes, irritants and allergens.

Verdict: Do not use soaps, commercial hand washes or soap-free bars. Look for natural liquid hand soaps that are 'sulfate-free' and preferably a plain unscented formula (available from health food shops). There are also sensitive skin liquid hand soaps available at most pharmacies — look for ones that are sulfate-free and with a pH range of 5 to 6.

Body washes

Body washes usually come in 'liquid soap' form that foams when friction is applied. Babies with eczema do not generally need to be washed with a body wash as it may irritate their eczema. If necessary, use sensitive skin body washes to cleanse under the arms and feet, and wash dirty hands.

Verdict: Use with caution. Look for products that are labelled 'sulfate-free' containing no sodium *lauryth* sulfate or sodium *lauryl* sulfate, and with a balanced pH of 5 to 6. These products should be low foaming or non-foaming.

Facial cleansers

Cleansers are used to dislodge dirt, pollution and make-up. The risk with using a foaming cleanser is that it may contain ingredients that strip the skin's natural oils, giving your skin a 'squeaky clean' effect. If your skin feels tight and dry after cleansing then the product is too harsh. A good cleanser can remove dirt and pollution without stripping your skin of all of its protective sebum.

Verdict: Look for non-foaming cleansers labelled 'sulfate-free' that feel creamy, not soapy, and that are non-bubbly when applied to the skin. Pure almond oil or jojoba oil can be used to remove make-up and, like all products, discontinue use if an adverse reaction occurs.

Toners

A well-designed toner can help to restore the natural acidic pH of the skin. However, toners can cause skin irritations so do not apply them to eczema or sensitive skin.

Verdict: Skip the toner in your beauty routine and spend your money on a good moisturiser instead.

Make-up

Make-up can have a place in your skin care routine if you choose. Be aware that all products deteriorate over time and bacteria from your fingers can contaminate make-up products and this might infect your eczema. As a general rule, make-up should be replaced within three years after leaving the factory. Natural make-up products that use natural preservatives, such as herbs, will have a shorter use-by-date so if using these products refer to the packaging for further details (there will probably be a symbol of a container with an opened lid and below it a reference to how many months it will last once opened). When a product deteriorates, you might see mould or a change in texture, consistency and/or smell. Avoid natural products that don't use preservatives as there is an increased risk of bacterial contamination when you have eczema or broken skin.

Make-up use-by-dates are shown in the table overleaf.

Cleaning your brushes and applicators

When you have broken skin, hygiene is very important, so wash your make-up brushes and other applicators once a week to remove bacteria.

Product	Estimated shelf life after opening	FYI (for your information)
Mascara	3–6 months	The pumping action can push bacteria to the bottom of the container
Moisturiser	3–12 months (refer to packaging)	Fingers dipped into a moisturiser tub can hasten bacterial contamination; enclosed pump or pourable containers are best
Cleanser	6–12 months (refer to packaging)	Use a non-foaming cleanser containing anti-inflammatory oils, p. 126
Blusher and eye shadow	1–2 years	Wash brushes regularly using hand soap and warm water
Facial powder, eyeliner, lipstick and lip liner	2 years	Don't share make-up
Foundation and concealer	12–18 months	Fingers can hasten bacterial contamination

Exfoliators

Exfoliating scrubs are creams and gels that contain granules or beads which dislodge skin flakes and smooth roughness. Do not use sharp scrubs made with crushed apricot kernels and don't exfoliate on or near eczema-affected areas or pimple-prone areas as this can cause irritation and spread infection. It's best to avoid exfoliators and body scrubs while you have eczema.

Deodorants and antiperspirants

Deodorants are body sprays that use fragrance, alcohol and chemicals to mask body odour. Antiperspirants can contain chemicals, parabens and aluminium and work by affecting the sweat gland to prevent sweating.

Verdict: Avoid chemical antiperspirants and use 'sensitive skin' deodorants when necessary: for example, if exercising or in hot weather. Most days, opt for a natural mineral salt deodorant (they look like a shaped crystal or a smooth salt rock). When moistened and rubbed under your arms, the minerals stop odour-causing bacteria. They are free of aluminium, are hypoallergenic and are fragrance- and paraben-free.

If you have eczema in your armpits avoid all forms of deodorants and use a moisturiser and dietary changes to improve your symptoms.

Sunscreen

It is important to protect eczema from excess sun exposure as sunburn can cause skin damage. However, in sensitive individuals, sunscreens can cause irritation if applied directly onto eczema. If using sunscreen, favour 'sensitive skin' sunscreens formulated for children and babies (as they are generally lower in chemicals than regular sunscreens) and avoid sunscreens that are artificially coloured.

Verdict: Protect your skin with clothing and a hat and apply sunscreen on unaffected areas.

Some sun exposure, free of sunscreen, is necessary for healthy skin and 10 minutes of direct sunlight on the skin daily is enough to prevent vitamin D deficiency.

Q & A: How to patch-test a skin care product

Q: 'I've tried eczema creams before and they always sting my skin. How do I know if a skin product is right for me?'

A: Test all skin care products on undamaged skin first. When testing an emollient, if your skin swells, burns or feels hot, tingly or slightly more irritated on undamaged skin then the moisturiser is not right for you. If your skin peels or flakes then the product is not suitable for you either. If a reaction occurs wash the product off and apply something soothing such as plain ointment.

If no reaction occurs after testing a product on undamaged skin then apply a small amount of moisturiser to one patch of your eczema. As your skin is damaged, this is likely to sting. Stinging may last between 1–3 minutes and you should stop reacting to a cream *within three applications*. For example, if you apply the moisturiser twice a day, then by the end of the second day your skin shouldn't sting at all. If your skin continues to hurt after the fourth application then you are probably reacting to an ingredient and you should wash the emollient off and discontinue use.

Skin care daily regime

Here is an example of a simple face cleansing regime for morning and evening.

Morning

- Wash hands with a gentle hand wash to remove bacteria, then rinse with water.
- Have a brief warm shower or bath for 5 to 10 minutes. Add oil to the bath if desired (see Chapter 9, 'Bath recipes + emergency itch busters'). Alternatively, fill a basin or large bowl with warm water and splash your face four to six times.
- After wetting your skin, gently pat with a soft cotton towel until your skin is nearly, but not quite, dry.
- Immediately apply a suitable emollient/moisturiser to your skin.

Note: If you cleansed your face the night before, then you don't need to use a cleanser in the morning; it's better to avoid over-cleaning your face so that your natural oils can work their magic.

Evening

- Wash your hands to remove bacteria, then rinse with water.
- Have a brief warm shower or bath for 5 to 10 minutes. Add oil to the bath if desired (see Chapter 9, 'Bath recipes + emergency itch busters'). Alternatively, fill a basin or large bowl with warm water and splash your face and neck four to six times.
- If you are removing make-up or have been exercising or have soiled skin, use a non-foaming cleanser and gently pat it onto your face and neck (babies and children do not need cleanser but they might occasionally need a gentle children's wash that is free of harsh ingredients — see 'Body washes' p. 126).
- Then, if cleansing, wet a cotton pad or ball or use a very soft facial cloth and gently wipe off the cleanser, pollution and make-up (if relevant).
- Thoroughly rinse off the cleanser with warm water.

- Gently pat your skin with a soft cotton towel until your skin is almost dry. Immediately apply a suitable emollient.

Key points to remember

When you have eczema it's essential to keep your skin care regime simple and avoid using topical products that can irritate the skin. Always read the label carefully and check the ingredients before buying products for your skin.

Chapter 8

General recommendations for eczema

While you have eczema, there are many ways to minimise your discomfort. Some of the following information is age-specific, so take from this list what is relevant to you in regards to age and living arrangements. This chapter ends with some information on what to do if your eczema becomes infected.

Create a healthy home

The environment you live in can irritate sensitive skin, however changes can be made to create an eczema-safe home, such as the following:

- Avoid mould — place moisture absorbers in all damp areas (these are available from hardware stores).
- Avoid cigarette smoke.
- Avoid using electric heating or airconditioning as they dry out the skin (if this is not possible, frequently apply an emollient to minimise moisture loss).
- Avoid pesticide and chemical exposures: farms that use crop spraying, living on a busy/polluted road, chemical cleaning products, nail polish containing formaldehyde, new carpets, new cars and new home and office furniture all release chemicals.

Healthy alternatives

Favour natural cleaning products (there are natural cleaning product recipes on p. 251). If you live on a farm or near an area that uses crop spraying, or on a busy/polluted road, ensure you eat a variety of alkalising eczema-safe vegetables and take antioxidants as these help the liver detoxify the chemicals you are being exposed to.

Ventilate the house by opening the windows each day as this will help to disperse chemicals released from furnishings.

Use eczema-safe bedding and fabrics

While you have broken skin you may be sensitive to dust mites and some types of fabrics. Ways to minimise discomfort include the following:

- Change bed linen weekly.
- Wash sheets in hot water or use a dryer to kill the dust mites.
- Take off tags from clothing as they can irritate the skin.
- Use 100 per cent cotton bedding.
- Avoid using doonas/duvets because they cause overheating (and eczema sufferers heat up quickly).
- Use woollen 'breathable' blankets in winter (but don't let woollen blankets touch the skin as they can cause irritation; ensure cotton sheets are long so they completely cover blankets).
- Dress in 100 per cent cotton clothing.
- Clothing can be worn inside out so the seams don't irritate babies with eczema.
- Wash clothing in sensitive skin or 'allergy' washing powder and avoid fabric softeners.

Improve sleep

Eczema sufferers benefit from having a sound night's sleep. To promote sleep, try the following:

- Avoid overtiredness (go to bed early rather than late).
- Laugh before bedtime. Funny films are useful in treating night-time waking in children with eczema according to research by Dr Hajime Kimata from the Department of Pediatrics and Allergy at the Ujitakeda Hospital in Kyoto, Japan. The benefit may be attributed in part to changes in the hormone level of ghrelin, which stimulates hunger. Compared to healthy children, salivary ghrelin levels are significantly elevated in patients with atopic eczema (which may

make them feel hungry at bedtime or during the night). Research shows that viewing a humorous film before bedtime lowers their salivary ghrelin levels and, as a result, children with eczema can experience a more restful night's sleep.[1]

- Melatonin, the hormone that promotes proper sleep, is often lower in eczema sufferers compared with healthy people and eczema sufferers can experience disturbed sleep as a result. Dr Kimata reports that watching a funny film increases melatonin production. In breastfeeding women, laughter increases melatonin in their breastmilk.[2]

A note on vaccinations

Vaccinating your child is a personal choice and I do not wish to advise you to be for or against it. If your child has eczema here are some basic facts to consider:

- Catching the measles or having vaccinations for measles, mumps and rubella (MMR) can trigger the appearance of atopic dermatitis, according to several research studies.[3] This may be related to nutritional deficiencies such as vitamin C. Studies show that vitamin C is depleted after receiving vaccinations, causing blood histamine levels to markedly increase and this can cause adverse symptoms. Taking vitamin C before and after vaccinations may assist with recovery, and babies on solids can be fed vitamin C-rich papaya.
- Some vaccines such as MMR vaccines and the flu vaccine contain traces of egg so if your child has an allergy to egg mention this to your doctor as there are egg-free alternatives.[4]
- Immunisations can and do save lives when outbreaks occur.
- Some doctors advise delaying immunisations if a child is unwell or has atopic eczema.

If you are concerned about vaccinating your child, please seek further information from your doctor.

Infected eczema: symptoms, care + prevention

Having eczema can sometimes make you feel as if you are sitting on top of an ant's nest, waiting for the ants to leave. And sometimes you just end up scratching even though you know you shouldn't. Scratching causes broken skin and an increased risk of bacterial, viral and fungal skin infections, school sores (impetigo) and cold sores (herpes simplex type 1) — all are good reasons to avoid scratching your skin!

Infections can also delay the healing of eczema so it's important to identify and treat them early. How do you know if your skin has become infected? It's sometimes difficult to spot an infection but *if your eczema suddenly worsens and does not respond to topical treatments* you should suspect an infection and immediately see your doctor. Also refer to the following list of symptoms.

Symptoms of infected eczema

Note that not all of these signs will be present at one time:

- hot and sore skin that is red and angry
- weepy/yellowish crust
- pus
- folliculitis (small red spots around the body hairs)
- tender, swollen glands in the neck, groin or armpits
- candida/fungal infection signs: red, itchy and sore skin and possibly tiny yellow pustules; white patches on the skin
- school sores (impetigo)
- cold sores (herpes simplex type 1)
- Eczema herpeticum signs: small blisters containing clear fluid or yellow pus, which break open and ulcerate; high temperature; general unwell feeling.

Infection care

If you suspect you have an infection see a doctor or visit your local hospital emergency room. Your doctor can do a fast and painless swab test to help identify the cause of the infection. Swabs help to identify which prescription would be most effective at eradicating the infection before it spreads and becomes dangerous. For example, the test may reveal the skin is infected with the bacteria *Staphylococcus aureus* or streptococci and these would require a vastly different treatment to a candida/fungal infection. By quickly treating your skin with the most appropriate medication, the infection should rapidly clear up.

Prevention

Even when you take the best care of your skin, it's not always possible to prevent eczema from becoming infected. However, you can reduce the risk of skin infections by following these guidelines.

Preventing infection in eczema

- ❋ The Eczema Diet boosts the immune system and promotes healthy skin barrier function so it can reduce the risk of infection.
- ❋ Avoid scratching itchy skin and minimise the itch by consuming alkalising foods and drinks.
- ❋ Do not share towels and face cloths/washers with other family members, especially if they have an infection such as a cold sore.
- ❋ Protect the skin's barrier and reduce dryness and cracking with daily use of moisturising creams and bath oils.
- ❋ Avoid soaps and dehydrating environments (such as airconditioning and heating) that dry out the skin and increase the risk of skin cracking.
- ❋ Avoid using unpreserved skin care products (preservatives prevent bacterial growth in a skin care product).
- ❋ Wash your hands frequently with a gentle hand soap (especially before applying emollients to your eczema).
- ❋ Avoid using old or out-of-date skin care products.
- ❋ Avoid using old or out-of-date make-up.

Chapter 9

Bath recipes + emergency itch busters

Bathing can be a useful way to temporarily relieve dry, itchy skin and adding oil to the water coats the skin and can help to lock in moisture. Depending on the severity of your eczema, keep the bath warm and under 10 minutes in duration so you don't dry out your skin. After bathing, pat your skin semi-dry with a soft towel then apply a suitable moisturiser. When choosing a bath oil look for ingredients such as evening primrose oil, emu oil, jojoba oil and borage oil. Avoid any bath products that bubble or contain sulfates.

How hot?

When bathing babies and children check the water temperature beforehand. It can be misleading using your hand to test the temperature of bath water as the skin on the palms is tougher than the rest of your body. To test if bath water is at a suitable temperature, put your elbow into the water. The bath water should not feel uncomfortably hot or too cold.

These recipes are for a standard-sized bath, filled one-third with water. Adjust the measurements according to the depth and size of your bath.

Bicarb Bath Recipe

THIS RECIPE IS ESPECIALLY USEFUL FOR BABIES AND IT CAN TEMPORARILY RELIEVE THE ITCH.

Add ¼ cup bicarbonate of soda (baking soda) to warm bath water and bathe for 5–10 minutes.

Moisturising Bath Recipe

EVENING PRIMROSE OIL IS USED AS AN EXAMPLE IN THESE RECIPES, HOWEVER, YOU CAN TEST A RANGE OF OILS TO SEE WHICH ONE IS BEST FOR YOUR SKIN.

1 teaspoon evening primrose oil or oil of choice (for a child's bath: 1 capsule, pierced)

1 tablespoon of your favourite emollient/moisturiser

Mix ingredients together (the moisturiser helps the oil to diffuse more easily) and then disperse it into a warm bath. Bathe for 5–10 minutes.

Salt Bath Recipe

Bathing in the ocean can help promote healing of the skin so if you live near the sea (and can brave the sting), have a swim. Alternatively, have a salt bath using Epsom salts which are rich in magnesium. This salt bath is mild but it still may sting. This recipe is suitable for adults.

¼ cup Epsom salts

¼ cup sea salt (use less if desired)

Add the salts to a warm bath and briefly dissolve the crystals. Soak for 10 minutes. Rinse off the salt with water, pat the skin semi-dry and moisturise immediately.

Emergency itch busters

The following are some natural, non-medical treatments that you can use at home when an itch attack occurs.

- Drink an alkalising drink to decrease acid in the body (acid in the tissues can cause itchiness). For example, drink a large glass of Tarzan Juice with added beetroot, p. 222, or eat a salad containing mung bean sprouts such as Alkaline Bomb Salad, p. 233.
- Take a supplement containing magnesium, glycine, vitamin C, vitamin B6 and calcium. Read more on eczema supplements in Chapter 6.
- Fill a plastic bag with ice cubes and hold it next to the skin.
- Have a bath using the Bicarb Bath Recipe, p. 137. Immediately after bathing, pat the skin until semi-dry then apply moisturiser to your entire body and, if necessary, sparingly apply an ointment over the itchy areas.

Chapter 10

Dandruff

Dandruff and seborrheic dermatitis are flaking, itchy skin conditions that affect more than 50 per cent of adults at some point in their life.[1] With dandruff, the flakes are usually oily and shed easily from the scalp. Seborrheic dermatitis is a more severe skin condition with the addition of inflammation and greasy, yellowish flakes which can be found on the scalp, ears, eyebrows, neck, chest and creases at the sides of the nose. Dandruff can occur when you have an oily scalp, if you are run down or stressed and it can occur in conjunction with psoriasis and eczema. Newborn babies who develop cradle cap, which shows up as thick yellow crusts on the scalp, can develop dandruff later in life.

While dandruff and seborrheic dermatitis appear when you have an oily scalp and altered microflora, these conditions do not occur on everyone. *Susceptible* people are at an increased risk of dandruff or seborrheic dermatitis because they have one or a combination of the following:

- nutritional deficiencies and/or excess sugar and starch in the diet (sugar feeds fungus/yeasts)
- a predisposition to other skin conditions such as cradle cap during childhood, psoriasis or eczema
- poor immunity (lowered defence against fungus/*Malassezia* proliferation)
- use of medical drugs
- neurotransmitter abnormalities
- damaged skin barrier/skin permeability (eczema!)
- immune response and allergic reactions triggered by *Malassezia* fungus/yeasts.[2]

Hair care practices can affect the health of the scalp and increase the risk of dandruff. This includes:

- hair product chemicals such as sulfates, which are typically found in shampoos (see the sulfate information on p. 122)
- excess use of hairspray or gel
- use of hair dyes
- infrequent shampooing
- inadequate rinsing of hair after washing
- pH changes in the scalp or skin (disrupted acid mantle/using hair cleansing products that are alkaline).

Microflora changes in the scalp

The composition of scalp microflora is altered in people with dandruff and seborrheic dermatitis.[3] Your immune system normally guards your skin from invading bacteria and yeasts but when you're run-down, stressed or not feeding your body correctly, your immune system can let its guard down. A common yeast called *Malassezia* (formerly called *Pityrosporum*) lives on the scalp and your immune system ensures that this freeloader doesn't multiply or claim too much territory. If your immune system fails to do its job, *Malassezia's* offspring, cousins, aunts and uncles take over your head and inflame your skin. *Malassezia* yeasts can be found on everyone but they flourish and cause dandruff in approximately 20 per cent of people. Research shows that people with dandruff have 74 per cent of the total microflora on their scalp as *Malassezia* and individuals with seborrheic dermatitis have 83 per cent as *Malassezia*. In contrast, people with healthy scalps (no dandruff) have only 46 per cent of the total microflora on their scalp as *Malassezia* yeasts.

On healthy scalps where there is no dandruff present, approximately 26 per cent of the microflora is *Corynebacterium acnes*, a non-pathogenic bacteria, but it reduces to 6 per cent in dandruff sufferers, and only 1 per cent in seborrheic dermatitis patients.[4]

A 3-step anti-dandruff plan

There are three basic steps to treat and prevent dandruff.

Step 1: Swap your shampoo

Shampoos can alter the scalp's pH, as can the use of gels, hairspray and hair dyes. Swap your sulfate-containing shampoo for a gentle shampoo (note that some natural shampoos can aggravate dandruff so you may need to try a few brands). There are a number of shampoo ingredients that are anti-fungal, anti-microbial and/or anti-inflammatory, including:

- tea tree oil*
- apple cider vinegar
- vitamin E
- panthenol (vitamin B5).

(*In a study, patients with dandruff were given either a shampoo with 5 per cent tea tree oil or a placebo shampoo. They were told to wash their hair daily, leaving the shampoo on for 3 minutes before rinsing. At the end of 4 weeks scalp lesions were significantly lower and less itching was seen in the tea-tree-oil shampoo users.)

Step 2: Spray your scalp

There is an anti-dandruff remedy you can make at home. This recipe is for the scalp only.

Daily Scalp Spray

This treatment can be applied before bed. If desired, you can wash it off in the morning. Use a quality spray bottle as cheap plastic may buckle from the vinegar.

1 medium spray bottle

½ teaspoon tea tree oil

6 drops pure vitamin E oil

6 teaspoons (30ml) apple cider vinegar (not double strength)

Fill the bottle with water, add the tea tree oil, vitamin E and apple cider vinegar, close the lid and shake well. Separate hair into sections so you can spray more directly onto the scalp. Spray your scalp. Dry your hair and style as usual. Lightly spray onto the scalp once a day or as necessary.

Step 3: Eat a healthy diet

Follow the Eczema Diet to help promote a strong immune system. Part 3 will cover everything you need to know, including recipes, menus and shopping guides, to get started on the Eczema Diet.

Chapter 11
Cradle cap

Cradle cap is a form of scalp dermatitis. It's not caused by poor hygiene and it's not contagious. The sebaceous glands in the infant's skin become inflamed and produce excess oil, which traps the skin as it sheds, forming thick yellow crusts on the scalp. Cradle cap predominantly affects babies during their first few months of life, however, if untreated, it can persist until the age of three and, very rarely, beyond three years. Unlike eczema, cradle cap is not itchy and it does not usually cause babies discomfort.

Symptoms and causes of cradle cap

The symptoms of cradle cap, as seen on the scalp, include:
- reddening of the skin
- greasy scalp
- thick yellow crusts that look like scabs/scales/flakes
- mild discomfort
- mild hair loss
- inflammation with small blisters that eventually pop and weep
- your child might become unwell.

Cradle cap can be caused by a number of factors, including:
- genetics (blood relatives are likely to have eczema and/or asthma)
- overactive sebaceous glands (from maternal hormones)
- it may appear in conjunction with seborrheic dermatitis (elsewhere on the body).

Treatment: if a skin infection is suspected see your doctor.

Cradle cap management

This is a two-step management plan for babies and children with cradle cap.

Step 1: Use gentle skin care

Hair: Find a natural baby shampoo that is free of sulfates (see the sulfate information on p. 122). Be suspicious if a children's product foams and bubbles. Also avoid coloured bath and skin products containing synthetic dyes and fragrances. You might need to visit your local health food shop to find a gentle baby shampoo (check the ingredients as some health food shops stock 'natural' and 'gentle' products that contain sodium lauryth sulfate). Gently shampoo your bub's hair and scalp often to gently remove the cradle cap.

Body: Note that it is not essential to wash your baby's body with foaming cleansers or soaps as this can disrupt the pH of their skin. Babies can be adequately cleaned with water and a very soft cloth.

Step 2: Use oil

Use a suitable oil to massage your baby's head, every second day if necessary (you can do this when you're bathing him/her). Then loosen the crusts by brushing the scalp, in a circular motion, with a very soft toothbrush or you can gently use a fine *plastic* toothcomb (not a metal one). Shampoo afterwards to remove most of the oil.

Suitable oils

To loosen the flakes you can use oils such as:

- calendula oil (diluted within a baby oil product)
- flaxseed oil (can be used on its own)
- evening primrose oil (can be used on its own)
- natural vitamin E (diluted within a baby oil product).

First patch-test the oil on unbroken skin and wait 24 hours to see if a reaction occurs. *Note:* Do not use products containing mineral oil, and keep all oils out of children's reach.

Part 3

Programs, menus + recipes

Health comes from within, from a body that is nourished and valued. Beauty follows.

Chapter 12

Getting started

Part 1 is the theory. Part 2 is the non-diet information. And Part 3 is where the practical application begins. Here are some steps to get you started.

Step 1: Read Part 1

Before beginning the Eczema Diet it's highly recommended you read Part 1 and do the mini questionnaires in Chapter 2 to help you identify problem areas in your diet and environment. Part 1 begins on p. 9 and the first questionnaire is on p. 17.

If you have a baby with eczema, start by reading Chapter 13, 'Infants with eczema', and if you have a child with eczema, aged between one and seventeen years, read Chapter 14, 'Children's meal plans + lunch box menus'. Adults with eczema should have a look at the suggested adult/family menu and familiarise yourself with the 3-day Alkalising Cleanse starting on p. 184.

Step 2: Peek in the pantry

Before beginning the diet, check your pantry and fridge and compare it to the 'Eczema-safe shopping guide: Stage 1' on pp. 260–261. Photocopy the shopping guide and cross off anything you already have.

Do you have handy kitchen appliances?

Useful appliances and utensils include a salad spinner and a water filter jug (no need to install expensive water filters unless you want to). A food processor mixes muffins, grates vegetables and whips up tasty dips. It is quite important to have a juicer to make fresh vegetable juices as this will speed up skin recovery time (I've had eczema patients heal their eczema without the addition of juices so you may be fine without one, but juicing does speed up results).

Other appliances and kitchen gadgets you may need include beaters, measuring cups, measuring spoons, a basting/pastry brush, a 12-hole muffin tray, a large baking tray, saucepans, both a large and small non-stick frying pan and a large casserole or roasting dish/pan with a lid. You will probably have most of these already. If you already have a slow cooker or a pressure cooker you can use it to make soups, broth and casseroles if you choose (though it is not essential to have one).

Step 3: Start shopping

Photocopy the 'Eczema-safe shopping guide: Stage 1' on pp. 260–261, choose some recipes and go shopping. You may need to visit a health food shop to get some of the ingredients. Adults with eczema can do the 3-day Alkalising Cleanse so write down the ingredients for these recipes. You will need to buy your supplements before you begin the cleanse program.

Step 4: Make broth

You will make your life easier if you have a cooking day one or two days before you begin the diet. The Therapeutic Broth on p. 226 is a key recipe throughout this diet and you will need to allocate time to let it simmer and gather richness (6 hours+). Then you need to let it cool down overnight in the refrigerator so it's easy to remove all the fat from the top (if the fat is not totally removed it will sabotage your diet, so don't skip this step). The broth will stay fresh for up to six days so you may need to freeze the leftovers.

It is handy to freeze 1 tablespoon-sized portions in an ice-cube tray, covered in plastic wrap. Then you can run the back of the tray under hot water to release them when you require them in a recipe for your child's dinner and so on. The soups and casseroles all require 3 cups of Therapeutic Broth so you can freeze portions of 3 cups of broth in freezer-proof containers for later use (though if you are an adult doing the 3-day Alkalising Cleanse you will use up the broth within the three days).

Other useful recipes to make the day before

If you have a child with eczema you might want to bake some Pear Muffins for your child's lunch box (p. 249) and make Sesame-free Hummus (p. 220) — these two recipes are not essential to the diet but they are handy. Also soak some oats or quinoa grains at the end of day 3 in preparation for breakfast on day 4 (for breakfast on day 4 I recommend making Omega Museli, p. 214, or if you are gluten-intolerant try Quinoa Porridge, p. 216).

Tips to fast-track your results

1. It's a good idea to have a juicing machine so you can make Tarzan Juice (p. 222) or Healthy Skin Juice (p. 222) daily as they are key recipes designed to decrease acid in the body and reduce eczema and itchy skin. If you do not have a juicer, you can consume the Alkaline Bomb Salad instead (p. 233).

2. A supplement containing vitamin C, magnesium ascorbate, glycine, vitamin B6, magnesium, natural vitamin E, biotin, zinc, vitamin D3 and chromium can speed up results (refer to Chapter 6, 'Eczema supplements').

Chapter 13
Infants with eczema

While eczema can occur at any age, it typically appears shortly after birth, between two and six months of age, and more than half of all eczema sufferers show signs of eczema before their first birthday. The following information outlines three steps you can take to minimise your baby's discomfort and reduce symptoms, and includes introducing solids at the appropriate age.

Assessing baby's eczema

The health and family history of an eczema sufferer, even of a newborn baby, can highlight key problem areas such as susceptibility to fungal infections, chemical exposure, consumption of raw egg white by the mother during pregnancy and so on. Before beginning the program fill out the questionnaires throughout Chapter 2, starting on p. 14. Here is an example of how a baby with eczema can be assessed by compiling a health history.

Case study A

Oscar developed eczema at eight weeks old. At six months of age, when solids were introduced, his eczema spread over his entire body and the eczema on his face made him look as though he was 'badly burned'. When the family history details were collected it was noted the family lived in an area where sugar cane and banana plantations were regularly sprayed with pesticides. One week before Oscar's birth, his mother had been treated with antibiotics and anti-fungals, which were necessary to treat an infection and candida overgrowth before having a natural birth (this indicates the need for probiotics and foods for gastrointestinal health). During her pregnancy the mother's diet had included frequent consumption of raw egg white (whole-egg mayonnaise and small amounts of raw cake mix when baking). The mother experienced dry, itchy skin during this time but no rash was present. This indicates the need for a biotin supplement.

When she breastfed her baby she noticed he would regularly pull away and cried 'like he was in pain'. When the mother stopped consuming dairy products and eggs she noticed her baby fed more peacefully, and after the change in her diet his previously 'explosive' poos, which happened at every nappy change, ceased being runny and green and normalised to once a day.

While the family were on holidays Oscar was briefly treated with cortisone cream, which initially helped his eczema but then it worsened. Oscar had been previously treated with topical antibiotics and oral steroids, which caused his eczema to worsen, and his skin also had white patches on it so I recommended he be treated for fungal infection (oral and topical) before starting the Eczema Diet program. Then the mother and Oscar were to resume taking a probiotic supplement containing *Lactobacillus rhamnosus* GG (Oscar was to have a few grains by mouth). His mother was asked to stop taking her breastfeeding multi supplement and was prescribed a supplement to increase glycine, magnesium, biotin, vitamins C, D and E and calcium in her breastmilk. The nutrients were chosen to help Oscar's liver deal with the chemical/pesticide load from his environment and to supply nutrients for the mother's health during breastfeeding (only the mother was to take the supplement, the baby received the nutrients second-hand through the breastmilk).

Oscar's mother also took flaxseed oil for omega-3 and she finished taking fish oil capsules (as her baby had not been tested for fish allergy these were not resumed). Oscar's mother changed her diet to eczema-safe foods and she consumed low-salicylate alkalising vegetable juices daily. As Oscar had recently started solids, a range of eczema-safe vegetables were added to his solids routine. Then meat was to be introduced to help boost iron consumption.

The update from a later consultation: Oscar's eczema improved but it was still present on his face and legs. As the baby's eczema worsened with the introduction of baby rice cereal at six months of age, the mother took rice out of their diets, and two weeks later Oscar's eczema completely cleared up from his face. He is now eczema-free.

Baby's milk + first foods

While your baby's only food source is milk (either breastmilk or formula), you have several ways to modify what types of nutrients he or she receives.

Breastfeeding

When you are breastfeeding, the nutrients from your diet pass into the breastmilk and then your child's body uses these nutrients for growth, repair and maintenance. While you are breastfeeding, you can modify your diet to change the nutrient composition in your milk so it is rich in anti-inflammatory and histamine-lowering nutrients. You can also avoid consuming the foods that are known to exacerbate eczema. To do this eat eczema-safe foods and avoid all other foods for a short period of time (approximately three months), and take the recommended eczema supplements. Note that the baby is not to be directly given these supplements (unless it is a suitable probiotic), and breastfeeding mothers are not to do the 3-day Alkalising Cleanse or go hungry (see 'Eczema-safe shopping guide: Stage 2', pp. 262–263, if extra variety is required). Ensure you're consuming plenty of eczema-safe vegetables, protein, grains, vitamin-C rich papaya and hydrating liquids. If you have a colicky or 'windy' baby you may also need to avoid garlic, leeks and spring onions (scallions). Use the 'Eczema-safe shopping guide: Stage 1', pp. 260–261.

Infant formula

If your baby is drinking infant formula, speak to your paediatrician or doctor about changing your baby to a low-allergy, non-dairy formula.

Probiotics

Probiotic supplements can be suitable for infants. See p. 113 for probiotic information.

Starting solids

Solids is the term used for the first foods you feed your baby and these foods are mushy and puréed to a smooth paste rather than being solid. Recent research shows that delaying the introduction of solids for more than six months can *increase* the risk of allergy and eczema so the current recommendation is to *start your baby on solids after four months of age*, unless advised otherwise by your paediatrician or doctor.[1] This general recommendation may not be suitable for all babies. Your baby needs to be able to sit upright while eating and if your baby is not showing signs of being ready for solids you can delay introducing solids for up to six months.

To identify allergies and intolerances, introduce each new food on its own and then continue with that food for three days before introducing the next food. It is a good idea to introduce new foods earlier in the day, rather than at bedtime (as once they're in bed you can't see if they are having an adverse reaction) — that way, if your child has a life-threatening anaphylactic reaction, where they have swelling and difficulty in breathing, you can spot it early and seek medical advice from a hospital or doctor. If your baby has a milder adverse reaction such as a flare-up, unsettled behaviour, diarrhoea* or vomiting*, keep a record in a diet diary and discontinue use of that particular food (you may want to re-test the food when your child is older). Avoid giving your baby foods they can choke on such as nuts, biscuits, toast and solid pieces of fruit or vegetables etc. (*Diarrhoea and vomiting can cause dehydration and hydrating electrolytes may be required. Seek your doctor's advice if this occurs.)

Commercial baby foods

Canned or jar baby foods are generally not recommended as they may contain ingredients that worsen eczema symptoms; however, if it is a plain variety (e.g. plain potato or plain stewed pear) then it may be suitable on occasion or as a 'back-up' option. If using commercial baby food, check that all ingredients are eczema-safe.

Foods from four months

Continue to feed your baby breastmilk or infant formula as usual. Then introduce the first food. In order of preference these are:

1. Plain baby rice cereal. Ensure it has added iron as a baby's iron stores begin to wane at this age. Choose plain varieties, no fruit flavours, and follow the packet instructions. If eczema symptoms worsen discontinue use and seek advice from a nutritionist. Quinoa may be a suitable alternative (but note it does not contain added iron).

2. Puréed vegetables. Eczema-safe vegetables are the best ones to try first. These include puréed white potato, sweet potato, carrot and choko

(chayote) (see 'Eczema-safe food charts: Stage 1', p. 253). If your child reacts to sweet potato or carrot they may be sensitive to salicylates.

3. Puréed fruit (vegies first, fruit second). Don't give your baby fruit before vegetables as they may develop a sweet tooth and reject savoury foods. Eczema-safe fruits are peeled puréed pear, mashed banana (not sugar variety), papaya and pawpaw (papaya is preferred). If your child reacts to banana, papaya or pawpaw they may be sensitive to amines.

It is essential that your baby consumes eczema-safe vegetables on a daily basis as vegetables will help your child to be eczema-free.

Foods from six months

Continue to give your baby rice cereal, eczema-safe vegetables and fruit, and infant formula and/or breastmilk during this time. Then add iron-rich meat and/or legumes to your baby's feeding routine as babies need extra iron in their diet for proper growth. When serving a baby meat, ensure the meat is very finely ground up and start with lean lamb and then try skinless chicken, both freshly minced (preservative-free, antibiotic-free, free range and/or organic is best, and it must be fresh). Then give mushy lentils, mashed chickpeas (garbanzo beans), mashed kidney beans and so on (refer to 'Eczema-safe shopping guide: Stage 1', pp. 260–261). Do not give your baby liver or lamb's fry as liver is the organ that can accumulate pesticides and chemicals.

Foods from eight months

If your baby is feeding well and ready for finger foods you can give him or her small slices of soft eczema-safe fruits, steamed soft carrot sticks, sweet potato and potato slices, and gluten-free rice or buckwheat pasta spirals (no corn/maize or wheat pastas, and no long spaghetti at this stage).

Foods from twelve months

Your child should be consuming chopped up foods by now to experience different textures and flavours. Refer to the next chapter for the children's meal plans.

Drinks

Best drinks for babies include breastmilk, non-dairy infant formula, pre-boiled water (see the box following) and Therapeutic Broth (p. 226). Once your child is six months old you can give them Tarzan Juice (p. 222) if desired (do not add mung bean sprouts to the juice as there is a risk of bacteria).

Sterilising baby's water

For children under the age of one year, water must be boiled to sterilise and kill bacteria, and then cooled before giving it to your baby. Do not give pre-boiled water to infants after the age of one, as your growing toddler's gastrointestinal tract needs to become accustomed to unsterilised water to challenge and strengthen their immune system. After the age of one, regular filtered water is recommended (filtered tap water).

Foods to avoid

Avoid giving your baby potentially problematic foods such as dairy products (cheese, yoghurt, butter, cow's milk etc.), eggs, fish and peanut butter and other nuts and pastes including tahini/sesame seed paste. Speak to your doctor about allergy testing before your child consumes these foods. Fruit juice, cordial and soft drink/sodas are not recommended for babies.

Teething

If your baby is teething you can make homemade rice rusks that are wheat- and dairy-free. They're easy to make and the recipe is on p. 224.

Teething gel

Avoid teething gels as they are rich in salicylates and can cause severe flare-ups in sensitive children. If you have a baby with eczema who is teething, you have a couple of options:

1. Use teething toys such as a freezable teething ring, which can be placed in the freezer and given to your child to chew on when the ring is cold.

2. If your child needs pain relief, you can talk to your doctor about using colour-free baby paracetamol: rub a very small amount onto your child's gums if he or she is unsettled because of teething pain.

General recommendations

- Make your child as comfortable as possible and use their prescribed medicated creams, if desired.
- To reduce the itch, refer to Chapter 9, 'Bath recipes + emergency itch busters'.
- If your child has a flare-up from a particular food, refer to the Eczema-safe food charts, p. 253, and see what chemical is present in that food.
- After your child turns one refer to Chapter 14, 'Children's meal plans +
- lunch box menus'.

Q & A: Immunisation

Q: 'What is the first thing I should feed my child after their immunisations?'

A: Before and after your child has vaccinations feed them papaya. Blood histamine levels elevate after immunisations, which can make a child appear unwell, and papaya is a rich source of histamine-lowering vitamin C. If you are breastfeeding, ensure you are taking vitamin C (a buffered form such as magnesium ascorbate or any ending in 'ascorbate' and vitamin B6 as they will pass through the breastmilk and can help your baby deal with the histamine influx caused by immunisations.

Chapter 14

Children's meal plans + lunch box menus

One in five children has eczema and, according to the National Eczema Society in the United Kingdom, there are no guarantees that a child will grow out of their eczema, although approximately 74 per cent are eczema-free by the age of sixteen. However, dietary changes can markedly speed up this process. This chapter outlines eczema-safe meal plans and lunch box menus for children aged one to seventeen years.

The following case study illustrates how a child with eczema can be assessed by compiling a complete health history.

Case study B

At fifteen months old Riley's eczema spread to most of his body so a complete health history was taken, which revealed the following: since three months of age Riley had suffered from eczema, both his parents suffer from hay fever and his aunt and uncle have asthma. His mother was managing Riley's eczema by moisturising him throughout the day, and he was given an antihistamine before bed if he was itchy and topical steroids were applied on the red patches. Riley's mother had already taken steps to make the house eczema-safe: she was ventilating the house daily and was already giving her child a suitable probiotic supplement for eczema.

Riley's eczema periodically worsens when he goes on long car trips (and if there is any change in routine) or if he eats foods he is allergic to or visits the family farm, where pesticides may be used. His eczema visibly worsens on hot and humid days, after swimming in chlorinated pools, after contact with grass or when crawling on carpet, sudden weather changes, on windy days and from stress. He always flares up for two weeks after receiving immunisations, which reveals his body may be slow at eliminating histamine from the blood (indicating the need for supplemental vitamin C, vitamin B6 and quercetin, and papaya in the diet). He has been allergy tested and is allergic to dairy, eggs, wheat, cod fish (other fish are okay), nuts, sesame seeds, latex and rye grass so he must avoid these. Riley had acid reflux for the first six months of life, which indicates he would benefit from alkalising foods in the diet (e.g. eczema-safe vegetables, banana, magnesium etc.) to promote acid–alkaline balance each day. He has shown no signs of fungal infection or candida overgrowth.

Riley's mother ate raw egg white (whole-egg mayonnaise and hollandaise sauce) once a month, before but not during pregnancy. The problematic foods in Riley's diet were watermelon, mangos, avocados, melon, passionfruit, mandarins, strawberries, jam, popcorn, Nuttelex™ (margarine), olive oil, broccoli, spaghetti bolognaise (tomato), corn/corn pasta and baked beans (these are rich in salicyaltes, natural MSG and the margarine is rich in omega-6). His mother was advised to avoid these and was given eczema-safe shopping lists, recipes and menus. A supplement was prescribed for Riley, which included biotin, glycine, magnesium, vitamin C, natural vitamin E, vitamin B12, folic acid, vitamin B6, zinc, vitamin D3, chromium, choline, inositol and calcium.

The update from Riley's mother three months after the initial consultation: Now that Riley is walking he does not flare up from carpet contact and a change in routine is not really a problem now. Within about two weeks of starting the Eczema Diet Riley's skin improved. Riley's skin has continued to improve, it remains clearer for longer and he doesn't get the all-over-body red rashes. Aside from Riley's allergy foods (dairy, eggs etc.), Riley's mother has reintroduced many of the foods but in moderation (once a week) and he seems to be fine with that.

The questionnaires in Chapter 2 can help you assess your child's eczema and compile a health history.

How many serves per day?

The following table can help you determine how many serves of each food type your child should be eating every day, depending on their age.

Age group	Wholegrains ✸ (oats, rice, spelt, barley, quinoa, buckwheat)	Vegetables ★ (eczema-safe + Tarzan Juice)	Fruit 🍎 (pear, banana, papaya, pawpaw)	Non-dairy milk and other ◗ (rice milk, oat milk, broth)	Protein/iron P (chicken, red meat, legumes, fish, beans, chickpeas)
1-3 yrs	1-2 serves (½-1 cup)	1-2 serves (½-1 cup)	1-2 serves (½-1 cup)	1-2 serves (½-1 cup)	½-1 serve (¼-½ cup)
4-7 yrs	2 serves (1 cup)	2-3 serves (1-1½ cups)	2 serves (1 cup)	2 serves (1 cup)	1 serve (½ cup)
8-17 yrs	2-3 serves (1-1½ cups)	3-4 serves (1½-2 cups)	2-3 serves (1-1½ cups)	2-3 serves (1-1½ cups)	1-2 serves (½-1 cup)

- For information on wholegrains see pp. 79–83.
- Stage 1 vegetables are: iceberg lettuce, cos (romaine) lettuce, mung bean sprouts, celery, cabbage (white or red), green beans, spring onions (scallions), potatoes (not desiree, sebago, pontiac, nardine), sweet potato (preferably not New Zealand kumera), carrots, swedes (rutabaga), fresh beetroot (not canned), parsley, chives, garlic (not Chinese), brussels sprouts, choko (chayote) and leeks.
- Eczema-safe fruits are peeled pear, banana (not sugar variety), papaya and pawpaw (the last three contain amines).
- Non-dairy milk: children with eczema should not consume dairy products so it is necessary to get your calcium from non-dairy sources which are fortified with calcium such as rice milk and from calcium-rich Therapeutic Broth (p. 226) which can be sipped warm during snack time or added to meals such as mashed potato and casseroles.
- Protein/iron: protein foods contain iron and both these nutrients are needed for healthy skin (see the protein information on pp. 83–87).

Iron

A child should eat two protein foods containing iron each day for growth. Iron sources from richest to poorest are: red meat, commercial rice or oat cereals with added iron, beans, lentils, wholemeal pasta, tofu, chicken, fish and wholemeal bread.

When you give your child a serve of iron-rich food, ensure it's not at the same time as consuming calcium-rich foods as calcium can prevent iron absorption and iron deficiency causes anaemia and slow growth. A child aged one to three years needs 9mg of iron daily. If you give your child two serves of protein-rich foods daily and wholegrains, they should consume enough iron.

Breakfast selection

Cereals can be served with rice milk, organic soy milk or oat milk.

- Omega Muesli, p. 214
- Surprise Porridge, p. 215, a puffed brown rice cereal or a plain puffed rice cereal
- Quinoa Porridge, p. 216
- Eczema-safe Fruit Salad, p. 217
- Buckwheat Crepes, p. 248
- Spelt Pancakes, p. 247
- spelt sourdough toast
- gluten-free bread with Banana Carob Spread, p. 220
- Spelt Lavash Bread, p. 229, with Banana Carob Spread, p. 220

Drink selection

- filtered water
- Tarzan Juice, p. 222
- Healthy Skin Juice, p. 222
- plain rice milk (calcium-fortified)
- Therapeutic Broth, p. 226 (serve warm)
- Healthy Skin Smoothie, p. 223
- Choco Milk, p. 245 (served warm or cold)
- pear water (from stewing peeled pears)

Snack selection

- carrot and celery sticks/shapes with Sesame-free Hummus, p. 220
- The Wishing Plate, p. 217
- sliced papaya

- peeled pear
- banana (not sugar variety)
- Pear Muffins, p. 249
- Spelt Lavash Bread, p. 229 (and spelt chips)
- Baked Banana Chips, p. 218
- plain rice crackers (no additives, no corn), with Bean Dip, p. 219
- plain rice cakes with Banana Carob Spread, p. 220
- Teething Rusks, p. 224
- wholegrain rye crispbread with Parsley Pesto, p. 221 (contains cashews)
- Potato Wedges, p. 218 (homemade)
- Banana Icy Poles, p. 245
- Banana on Sticks, p. 250
- stewed pear (reserve the water for drinks)

Lunch and dinner selection

- Design Your Own Sandwich, p. 228
- Spelt Lavash Bread, p. 229 with Banana Carob Spread, p. 220
- sliced roast chicken/lamb (home cooked, no artificial additives, fat drained)
- New Potato and Leek Soup, p. 234
- Papaya Rice Paper Rolls, p. 230
- Chickpea Casserole, p. 242 (can use chicken, lamb or fish)
- Chickpea Rice, p. 231 (optional: add chicken, lamb or fish)
- Roasted Potato Stack, p. 232
- Sunshine Soup, p. 235
- Baked Fish with Mash, p. 237
- Easy Roast Chicken, p. 240
- Country Chicken Soup, p. 236
- Cinnamon Chicken, p. 241 (omit cinnamon during Stage 1)
- Alkaline Bomb Salad, p. 233
- Sticks and Stones, p. 238
- Pasta, p. 244 (chicken, lamb, beans or fish)
- My Favourite Lamb Cutlets, p. 243

- lean lamb (fat removed), green beans and potatoes
- veal, carrots and Smashed Potato, p. 239

DIY suggestions

I encourage you to experiment with the eczema-safe ingredients and create your own meals, for example:

- lean lamb/chicken/fish/veal with green beans, brussels sprouts and Smashed Potato, p. 239
- lean lamb/chicken/fish/veal/beans with roasted carrots and Potato Wedges, p. 218
- grilled chicken served with Alkaline Bomb Salad, p. 233
- vegetarians and vegans: plain tofu with kidney beans, quinoa and diced carrots
- chicken casserole with potatoes, sweet potato, carrots, leeks and celery (modify Chickpea Casserole recipe, p. 242).

Must your child eat meat?

If you are vegetarian or vegan it is not necessary to eat red meat, fish or chicken during the Eczema Diet. Recipes containing meat are on the menu mainly for variety (and they supply protein and iron). Please choose vegetarian soups and eat beans if preferred. If a dinner recipe contains animal product and it cannot be converted to a vegetarian or vegan meal, then an option marked with 'V&Vn' will be given or there will be soup options. Many of the recipes in the menus are already suitable for vegetarians and vegans (such as breakfasts and snacks) and these are not marked with 'V&Vn'.

Avoid these: tempeh, vegan/vegetarian patties and sausages, and other meat substitutes as they can contain additives, soy sauce and/or natural flavourings and herbs.

Gluten intolerance

If your child cannot eat gluten, the gluten-free meals are marked with 'GF' in the recipe section and most meals can be converted to gluten-free.

Menus

The following food plans were designed for some of my young eczema patients. The menus are guides only: you'll need to adjust them to suit your child's age, allergies and appetite and ensure they consume protein, dietary fibre, liquids such as water and eczema-safe fruits and vegetables. The symbols ★ ●P◆ ✹ appear at the top of the menus as a reminder to give your child some vegies, fruit, wholegrains, protein or liquid at that particular meal. You don't have to strictly follow these suggestions, but if it becomes a habit for you to think 'Lunch time is when I serve wholegrains', or 'I'll serve protein with dinner', it will be easier to give your child a nutritious and balanced diet.

The following menus are free of wheat, dairy, nuts and eggs, and contain alkalising foods and drinks. Before you begin, read 'Chapter 12: Getting started', p. 145, and make Therapeutic Broth, p. 226, a full day or two before you start day 1, and you might want to freeze some whole bananas as they make great desserts (peel them and place them in a sealed container). You'll see there is a 'treat day' every seventh day and you can adapt this to suit your child so they have something to look forward to each week. Suggested meals are in the menus and you have several choices to choose from (also refer to the lists in this chapter and the 'Eczema-safe shopping guide: Stage 1', pp. 260–261).

Fussy eating habits

You'll see on the menus coming up shortly that there are phrases written near the top of some of the columns, such as 'time for eczema-safe vegies' and 'morning tea is fruit time'. These phrases are really effective tools to help guide a child to accept and enjoy a healthy eating program. If said daily, these phrases can help your child form new eating habits over a matter of days or weeks (for more tips on inspiring fussy kids to eat healthy foods refer to 'Resources' p. 265).

Rate your child's eczema

Before beginning the program, you can rate your child's eczema (refer to 'Rate your eczema', p. 188) and you may like to take photos of your child's eczema so you can document their skin condition before and after.

Day 0: __/ __/ ____   Skin condition: ____/10

Day 1

Breakfast ✹ ◉	Morning snack ◉	Lunch ✹
Supplements with Tarzan Juice, p. 222, filtered water or rice milk Choose from: Surprise Porridge, p. 215; Omega Muesli, p. 214; plain rice cereal with rice milk; or Quinoa Porridge, p. 216	'Morning tea is fruit time' Choose from: papaya, banana and/or pear; plain rice crackers; Pear Muffin, p. 249; Baked Banana Chips, p. 218; spelt pikelets with rice malt syrup and banana (use Spelt Pancakes recipe, p. 247); or Healthy Skin Smoothie, p. 223 Filtered water	'Brainy grain time' Choose from: Design Your Own Sandwich, p. 228; or Pasta with beans, chicken or fish, p. 244 Filtered water

Afternoon snack ★	Dinner P ★ ★	Rate your eczema: /10
'Afternoon tea is vegie time' Choose from: carrot and celery sticks, rice crackers and Sesame-free Hummus, p. 220 or Bean Dip, p. 219; Wishing Plate, p. 217; or Alkaline Bomb Salad, p. 233 Tarzan Juice, p. 222, Healthy Skin Juice, p. 222 or filtered water	Chickpea Casserole, p. 242, or soup of choice, pp. 234–236 Optional dessert: frozen banana slices, eczema-safe fruits, or Pear Muffin, p. 249 Filtered water or rice milk	Notes:

Day 2

Breakfast ❋ ◊	Morning snack ◉	Lunch ❋
Supplements with Tarzan Juice, p. 222, filtered water or rice milk Choose from: Surprise Porridge, p. 215; plain rice cereal with rice milk; Quinoa Porridge, p. 216; or Omega Muesli, p. 214	'Morning tea is fruit time' Choose from: papaya balls (use a melon baller), banana and/or pear; plain rice crackers; Pear Muffin, p. 249; Baked Banana Chips, p. 218; spelt pikelets with rice malt syrup and banana (use Spelt Pancakes recipe, p. 247); or Healthy Skin Smoothie, p. 223 Filtered water	'Brainy grain time' Choose from: Design Your Own Sandwich, p. 228; or Pasta with beans, chicken or fish, p. 244 Filtered water

Afternoon snack ★	Dinner P ★ ★	Rate your eczema: /10
'Afternoon tea is vegie time' Choose from: carrot and celery sticks, rice crackers and Sesame-free Hummus, p. 220 or Bean Dip, p. 219; or Alkaline Bomb Salad, p. 233 Tarzan Juice, p. 222 or filtered water	Choose from: New Potato and Leek Soup, p. 234 with gluten-free bread or Spelt Lavash Bread, p. 229, or use up leftovers Filtered water or rice milk	Notes:

Day 3

Breakfast ✳ ●

Supplements with Tarzan Juice, p. 222, filtered water or rice milk

Choose from: Surprise Porridge, p. 215; plain rice cereal with rice milk; Quinoa Porridge, p. 216; or Omega Muesli, p. 214 with Baked Banana Chips, p. 218 (or a banana)

Morning snack ●

'Morning tea is fruit time'

Choose from: papaya, banana and/or pear; plain rice crackers; Pear Muffin, p. 249; Baked Banana Chips, p. 218; spelt pikelets with rice malt syrup and banana (use Spelt Pancakes recipe, p. 247) or Healthy Skin Smoothie, p. 223

Filtered water

Lunch ✳

'Brainy grain time'

Choose from: Design Your Own Sandwich, p. 228; or Pasta with beans, chicken or fish, p. 244

Filtered water

Afternoon snack ★

'Afternoon tea is vegie time'

Choose from: carrot and celery sticks, rice crackers and Sesame-free Hummus, p. 220 or Bean Dip, p. 219; Wishing Plate, p. 217; or Alkaline Bomb Salad, p. 233

Tarzan Juice, p. 222 or filtered water

Dinner P ★ ★

Choose from: Cinnamon Chicken, p. 241 (don't use cinnamon in Stage 1); or use up leftover soup

Filtered water or rice milk

Rate your eczema: /10

Notes:

Day 4

Breakfast ❋ ♦	Morning snack 🍎	Lunch ❋
Supplements with Tarzan Juice, p. 222, filtered water or rice milk Choose from: Surprise Porridge, p. 215; plain rice cereal with rice milk; Quinoa Porridge, p. 216; or Omega Muesli, p. 214	'Morning tea is fruit time' Choose from: papaya, banana and/or pear; plain rice crackers; Pear Muffin, p. 249; Baked Banana Chips, p. 218; spelt pikelets with rice malt syrup and banana (use Spelt Pancakes recipe, p. 247); or Healthy Skin Smoothie, p. 223 Filtered water	'Brainy grain time' Choose from: Design Your Own Sandwich, p. 228 Filtered water

Afternoon snack ★	Dinner P ★ ★	Rate your eczema: /10
'Afternoon tea is vegie time' Choose from: carrot and celery sticks, rice crackers and Sesame-free Hummus, p. 220 or Bean Dip, p. 219; Wishing Plate, p. 217; or Alkaline Bomb Salad, p. 233 Tarzan Juice, p. 222, Healthy Skin Juice, p. 222 or filtered water	Choose from: Baked Fish with Mash, p. 237 or use up leftovers; or soup of choice, pp. 234–236 Filtered water or rice milk	**Notes:**

Day 5

Breakfast ✹ ◗	Morning snack 🍎	Lunch ✹
Supplements with Tarzan Juice, p. 222, filtered water or rice milk Choose from: Surprise Porridge, p. 215; plain rice cereal with rice milk; Quinoa Porridge, p. 216; or Omega Muesli, p. 214	'Morning tea is fruit time' Choose from: papaya, banana and/or pear; plain rice crackers; Pear Muffin, p. 249; Baked Banana Chips, p. 218; spelt pikelets with rice malt syrup and banana (use Spelt Pancakes recipe, p. 247); or Healthy Skin Smoothie, p. 223 Filtered water	'Brainy grain time' Choose from: Design Your Own Sandwich, p. 228; or Pasta with beans, chicken or fish, p. 244 Filtered water

Afternoon snack ★	Dinner P ★	Rate your eczema: /10
'Afternoon tea is vegie time' Choose from: carrot and celery sticks, rice crackers and Sesame-free Hummus, p. 220 or Bean Dip, p. 219; Wishing Plate, p. 217; or Alkaline Bomb Salad, p. 233 Tarzan Juice, p. 222, or filtered water	Choose from: Country Chicken Soup, p. 236, or Papaya Rice Paper Rolls, p. 230; or soup of choice, pp. 234–236 Optional dessert: frozen banana slices Filtered water or rice milk	Notes:

Day 6

Breakfast ✳ ◆

Supplements with Tarzan Juice, p. 222, filtered water or rice milk

Choose from: Surprise Porridge, p. 215; plain rice cereal with rice milk; Quinoa Porridge, p. 216; or Omega Muesli, p. 214

Morning snack 🍎

'Morning tea is fruit time'

Choose from: papaya, banana and/or pear; plain rice crackers; Pear Muffin, p. 249; Baked Banana Chips, p. 218; spelt pikelets with rice malt syrup and banana (use Spelt Pancakes recipe, p. 247) or Healthy Skin Smoothie, p. 223

Filtered water

Lunch ✳

'Brainy grain time'

Choose from: Design Your Own Sandwich, p. 228; or Pasta with beans, chicken or fish, p. 244

Filtered water

Afternoon snack ★

'Afternoon tea is vegie time'

Choose from: carrot and celery sticks, rice crackers and Sesame-free Hummus, p. 220 or Bean Dip, p. 219; Wishing Plate, p. 217; or Alkaline Bomb Salad, p. 233

Tarzan Juice, p. 222 or filtered water

Dinner P ★

Choose from: Sticks and Stones, p. 238 or use up leftovers; or soup of choice, pp. 234–236

Filtered water or rice milk

Rate your eczema: /10

Notes:

Day 7 Treat day

Breakfast ✹ ◐	Morning snack ◉	Lunch ✹
Supplements with Tarzan Juice, p. 222, filtered water or rice milk Choose from: Spelt Pancakes, p. 247; plain rice cereal with rice milk; Buckwheat Crepes, p. 248; or Healthy Skin Smoothie, p. 223	'Morning tea is fruit time' Choose from: papaya, banana and/or pear; Pear Muffin, p. 249; spelt pikelets with rice malt syrup and banana (use Spelt Pancakes recipe, p. 247); vanilla soy yoghurt (no 160b/annatto) with fresh pear; or Healthy Skin Smoothie, p. 223 Filtered water	'Brainy grain time' Choose from: Design Your Own Sandwich, p. 228; or Pasta with beans, chicken or fish, p. 244 Filtered water

Afternoon snack ★	Dinner P ★	Rate your eczema: /10
'Afternoon tea is vegie time' Choose from: carrot and celery sticks, rice crackers and Sesame-free Hummus, p. 220 or Bean Dip, p. 219; Wishing Plate, p. 217; or Alkaline Bomb Salad, p. 233 Tarzan Juice, p. 222, Healthy Skin Juice, p. 222 or filtered water	'Treat Sunday' Choose from: Easy Roast Chicken, p. 240 or soup of choice, pp. 234–236 Optional dessert: Banana on Sticks, p. 250; Banana Icy Pole, p. 245 or Spelt Pancakes, p. 247 Filtered water, rice milk or Choco Milk, p. 245	Notes:

Day 8

Breakfast ✹ ●	Morning snack 🍎	Lunch ✹
Supplements with Tarzan Juice, p. 222, filtered water or rice milk	'Morning tea is fruit time'	'Brainy grain time'
Choose from: Surprise Porridge, p. 215; plain rice cereal with rice milk; Quinoa Porridge, p. 216; or Omega Muesli, p. 214 with Baked Banana Chips, p. 218 (or a banana)	Choose from: papaya, banana and/or pear; multigrain rye crackers; Pear Muffin, p. 249; Baked Banana Chips, p. 218; spelt pikelets with rice malt syrup and banana (use Spelt Pancakes recipe, p. 247); or Healthy Skin Smoothie, p. 223	Choose from: Design Your Own Sandwich, p. 228; or Pasta with beans, chicken or fish, p. 244
		Filtered water
	Filtered water	

Afternoon snack ★	Dinner P ★	Rate your eczema: /10
'Afternoon tea is vegie time'	Choose from: Chickpea Rice, p. 231 (with leftover chicken) or use up leftovers; or soup of choice, pp. 234–236	Notes:
Choose from: carrot and celery sticks, rice crackers and Sesame-free Hummus, p. 220 or Bean Dip, p. 219; Wishing Plate, p. 217; or Alkaline Bomb Salad, p. 233	Filtered water or rice milk	
Tarzan Juice, p. 222, or filtered water		

Day 9

Breakfast ✹ ◆

Supplements with Tarzan Juice, p. 222, filtered water or rice milk

Choose from: Surprise Porridge, p. 215; plain rice cereal with rice milk; Quinoa Porridge, p. 216; Omega Muesli, p. 214 with Baked Banana Chips, p. 218 (or a banana)

Morning snack ◉

'Morning tea is fruit time'

Choose from: papaya, banana and/or pear; multigrain rye crackers; Pear Muffin, p. 249; Baked Banana Chips, p. 218; spelt pikelets with rice malt syrup and banana (use Spelt Pancakes recipe, p. 247); or Healthy Skin Smoothie, p. 223

Filtered water

Lunch ✹

'Brainy grain time'

Choose from: Design Your Own Sandwich, p. 228; or Pasta with beans, chicken or fish, p. 244

Filtered water

Afternoon snack ★

'Afternoon tea is vegie time'

Choose from: carrot and celery sticks, rice crackers and Sesame-free Hummus, p. 220 or Bean Dip, p. 219; Wishing Plate, p. 217; or Alkaline Bomb Salad, p. 233

Tarzan Juice, p. 222 or filtered water

Dinner P ★

Choose from: Sunshine Soup, p. 235; or My Favourite Lamb Cutlets, p. 243; or use up leftovers; or soup of choice, pp. 234–236

Dessert: papaya (rich in vitamin C to help iron absorption)

Filtered water or rice milk

Rate your eczema: /10

Notes:

Day 10

Breakfast ☀ ◉	Morning snack 🍎	Lunch ☀
Supplements with Tarzan Juice, p. 222, filtered water or rice milk Choose from: Surprise Porridge, p. 215; plain rice cereal with rice milk; Quinoa Porridge, p. 216; Omega Muesli, p. 214 with Baked Banana Chips, p. 218 (or a banana)	'Morning tea is fruit time' Choose from: papaya, banana and/or pear; multigrain rye crackers; Pear Muffin, p. 249; Baked Banana Chips, p. 218; spelt pikelets with rice malt syrup and banana (use Spelt Pancakes recipe, p. 247); or Healthy Skin Smoothie, p. 223 Filtered water	'Brainy grain time' Choose from: Design Your Own Sandwich, p. 228; or Pasta with beans, chicken or fish, p. 244 Filtered water

Afternoon snack ★	Dinner P ★	Rate your eczema: /10
'Afternoon tea is vegie time' Choose from: carrot and celery sticks, rice crackers and Sesame-free Hummus, p. 220 or Bean Dip, p. 219; Wishing Plate, p. 217; or Alkaline Bomb Salad, p. 233 Tarzan Juice, p. 222, Healthy Skin Juice, p. 222 or filtered water	Choose from: Chickpea Casserole, p. 224 or Papaya Rice Paper Rolls, p. 230; or soup of choice, pp. 234–236 Filtered water or rice milk	Notes:

Day 11

Breakfast ❋ ◉	Morning snack ◉	Lunch ❋
Supplements with Tarzan Juice, p. 222, filtered water or rice milk Choose from: Surprise Porridge, p. 215; plain rice cereal with rice milk; Quinoa Porridge, p. 216; Omega Muesli, p. 214 with Baked Banana Chips, p. 218 (or a banana)	'Morning tea is fruit time' Choose from: papaya, banana and/or pear; multigrain rye crackers; Pear Muffin, p. 249; Baked Banana Chips, p. 218; spelt pikelets with rice malt syrup and banana (use Spelt Pancakes recipe, p. 247); or Healthy Skin Smoothie, p. 223 Filtered water	'Brainy grain time' Choose from: Design Your Own Sandwich, p. 228; or Pasta with beans, chicken or fish, p. 244 Filtered water

Afternoon snack ★	Dinner P ★	Rate your eczema: /10
'Afternoon tea is vegie time' Choose from: carrot and celery sticks, rice crackers and Sesame-free Hummus, p. 220 or Bean Dip, p. 219; Wishing Plate, p. 217; or Alkaline Bomb Salad, p. 233 Tarzan Juice, p. 222, Healthy Skin Juice, p. 222 or filtered water	Choose from: Pasta, p. 244 or use up leftovers; or soup of choice, pp. 234–236 Filtered water or rice milk	Notes:

Day 12

Breakfast ✹ ◆

Supplements with Tarzan Juice, p. 222, filtered water or rice milk

Choose from: Surprise Porridge, p. 215; plain rice cereal with rice milk; Quinoa Porridge, p. 216; Omega Muesli, p. 214 with Baked Banana Chips, p. 218 (or a banana)

Morning snack 🍎

'Morning tea is fruit time'

Choose from: papaya, banana and/or pear; multigrain rye crackers; Pear Muffin, p. 249; Baked Banana Chips, p. 218; spelt pikelets with rice malt syrup and banana (use Spelt Pancakes recipe, p. 247); or Healthy Skin Smoothie, p. 223

Filtered water

Lunch ✹

'Brainy grain time'

Choose from: Design Your Own Sandwich, p. 228; or Pasta with beans, chicken or fish, p. 244

Filtered water

Afternoon snack ★

'Afternoon tea is vegie time'

Choose from: carrot and celery sticks, rice crackers and Sesame-free Hummus, p. 220 or Bean Dip, p. 219; Wishing Plate, p. 217; or Alkaline Bomb Salad, p. 233

Tarzan Juice, p. 222, Healthy Skin Juice, p. 222 or filtered water

Dinner P ★

Choose from: My Favourite Lamb Cutlets, p. 243; or use up leftovers; or soup of choice, pp. 234–236

Dessert: papaya (rich in vitamin C to help iron absorption)

Filtered water or rice milk

Rate your eczema: /10

Notes:

Day 13

Breakfast ✱ ◆

Supplements with Tarzan Juice, p. 222, filtered water or rice milk

Choose from: Surprise Porridge, p. 215; plain rice cereal with rice milk; Quinoa Porridge, p. 216; Omega Muesli, p. 214 with Baked Banana Chips, p. 218 (or a banana)

Morning snack 🍎

'Morning tea is fruit time'

Choose from: papaya, banana and/or pear; multigrain rye crackers; Pear Muffin, p. 249; Baked Banana Chips, p. 218; spelt pikelets with rice malt syrup and banana (use Spelt Pancakes recipe, p. 247); or Healthy Skin Smoothie, p. 223

Filtered water

Lunch ✱

'Brainy grain time'

Choose from: Design Your Own Sandwich, p. 228; or Pasta with beans, chicken or fish, p. 244

Filtered water

Afternoon snack ★

'Afternoon tea is vegie time'

Choose from: carrot and celery sticks, rice crackers and Sesame-free Hummus, p. 220 or Bean Dip, p. 219; Wishing Plate, p. 217; or Alkaline Bomb Salad, p. 233

Tarzan Juice, p. 222, or filtered water

Dinner P ★

Choose from: Baked Fish with Mash, p. 237 (use flathead or eczema-safe white fish, p. 72); or soup of choice, pp. 234–236

Filtered water or rice milk

Rate your eczema: /10

Notes:

Day 14 Treat day

Breakfast ✻ ◆	Morning snack 🍎	Lunch ✻
Supplements with Tarzan Juice, p. 222, filtered water or rice milk Choose from: Spelt Pancakes, p. 247; plain rice cereal with rice milk; Buckwheat Crepes, p. 248 (GF option) or Healthy Skin Smoothie, p. 223	'Morning tea is fruit time' Choose from: papaya balls (using a melon baller), banana and/or pear; Pear Muffin, p. 249; spelt pikelets with rice malt syrup and banana (use Spelt Pancakes recipe, p. 247); vanilla soy yoghurt (no 160b/annatto) with fresh pear; or Healthy Skin Smoothie, p. 223 Filtered water	'Brainy grain time' Choose from: Design Your Own Sandwich, p. 228; or Pasta with beans, chicken or fish, p. 244 Filtered water

Afternoon snack ★	Dinner P ★	Rate your eczema: /10
'Afternoon tea is vegie time' Choose from: carrot and celery sticks, rice crackers and Sesame-free Hummus, p. 220 or Bean Dip, p. 219; Wishing Plate, p. 217; or Alkaline Bomb Salad, p. 233 Tarzan Juice, p. 222, Healthy Skin Juice, p. 222 or filtered water	'Treat Sunday' Choose from: Easy Roast Chicken, p. 240 (or use a lean cut of lamb); or soup of choice, pp. 234–236 Optional dessert: Banana on Sticks, p. 250, Banana Icy Pole, p. 245, or Spelt Pancakes, p. 247 Filtered water, rice milk or Choco Milk, p. 245	Notes:

Lunch box menus

The following lunch box menus are designed for your child to eat either at home or to take with them to day care or school (the afternoon snack is there for consumption during long day care or after school). Each day there is a range of meals to choose from, keeping in mind the menus are a guide only and you will need to adjust the portion sizes to suit your child's age, appetite and feeding ability.

Don't forget!

Remember to pack: a water bottle; utensils such as a spoon or fork if packing yoghurt, salad, beans or tuna; a small freezer block to keep perishable protein items cold and fresh (such as yoghurt, fish, meat and soy). *There is an increased risk of food poisoning if these items aren't kept cool. Tip:* papaya is an important source of vitamin C and skin-protective lycopene so ideally your child should eat it daily.

Lunch box menu A (age 1–3 years)

Mid-morning snack	Lunch	Afternoon snack
Day 1		
Choose from: peeled pear; papaya; banana (not sugar variety), and/or Pear Muffin, p. 249 Water bottle (filtered water)	Design Your Own Sandwich, p. 228 or *gluten-free pasta spirals with lamb, kidney beans and soft carrot or green beans Pack a spoon and freezer block	Celery cut into 'shark's teeth' shapes (not sticks as they may be too chewy, see p. 217) and plain rice crackers or spelt chips (use Spelt Lavash Bread recipe, p. 229)
Day 2		
Choose from: papaya balls (use a melon baller); banana Water bottle (filtered water)	Design Your Own Sandwich, p. 228 or wheat-free sandwich with diced/sliced chicken (home-cooked or organic) with grated carrot or shredded iceberg lettuce. Pack a freezer block	Spelt chips (use Spelt Lavash Bread recipe, p. 229) and serve with Sesame-free Hummus, p. 220

Mid-morning snack	Lunch	Afternoon snack
Day 3		
Pear Muffin, p. 249; banana Water bottle (filtered water)	Design Your Own Sandwich, p. 228 or wheat-free sandwich with Banana Carob Spread, p. 220	'Shark's teeth' celery slices, and vanilla soy yoghurt (no 160b /annatto) with chopped canned pear and papaya Pack a spoon and freezer block
Day 4		
Choose from: peeled pear and papaya balls; plain rice cakes/crackers Water bottle (filtered water)	Design Your Own Sandwich, p. 228 or *'Potato Man' (kidney/green beans, carrot and/or celery slotted into a baked potato to make a 'potato man' — serve with extra kidney beans in an iceberg lettuce leaf 'cup') Pack a spoon and freezer block	Spelt chips (use Spelt Lavash Bread recipe, p. 229) and serve with Bean Dip, p. 219
Day 5 'Friday is treat day'		
Choose from: banana; peeled pear slices and celery cut into 'Shark's teeth' shapes (not sticks as they may be too chewy) Water bottle (filtered water)	Design Your Own Sandwich, p. 228 or wheat-free sandwich with Banana Carob Spread, p. 220	New Anzac Cookies, p. 250 and/or vanilla soy yoghurt (no 160b/annatto) topped with Banana Carob Spread, p. 220; or papaya and chopped canned pear Pack a spoon and freezer block

(*You can use dinner leftovers for lunch, and most of the recipes in Chapter 18 are suitable. Just be sure to adjust the portions and cut up foods into smaller bite-sizes to suit your child's age and feeding ability.)

Lunch box menu B (age 3+)

Mid-morning snack	Lunch	Afternoon snack
Day 1		
Choose from: peeled and sliced pear; papaya; plain rice cakes/crackers; and Baked Banana Chips, p. 218 Water bottle (filtered water)	Design Your Own Sandwich, p. 228 or *gluten-free pasta spirals with lamb, kidney beans and soft carrot or green beans Pack a spoon and freezer block	Carrot sticks with Sesame-free Hummus, p. 220 or Bean Dip, p. 219, and spelt chips (use Spelt Lavash Bread recipe, p. 229)
Day 2		
Choose from: papaya balls (use a melon baller); banana (not sugar variety); plain rice cakes/crackers Water bottle (filtered water)	Design Your Own Sandwich, p. 228 or wheat-free sandwich with thinly sliced chicken (home-cooked or organic) with shredded iceberg lettuce Pack a spoon and freezer block	Peeled celery sticks with Sesame-free Hummus, p. 220 (spread in groove), and spelt chips (use Spelt Lavash Bread recipe, p. 229).
Day 3		
Pear Muffin, p. 249 and a banana Water bottle (filtered water) Pack a freezer block	Design Your Own Sandwich, p. 228 or Papaya Rice Paper Rolls, p. 230	Plain rice crackers and peeled carrot sticks with Bean Dip, p. 219
Day 4		
Choose from: papaya; peeled pear (pack a fork); plain rice cakes/crackers Water bottle (filtered water)	Design Your Own Sandwich, p. 228 or *Potato salad with diced potato, kidney beans, celery and iceberg lettuce (and diced papaya for sweetness) Pack a spoon and freezer block	Spelt chips (use Spelt Lavash Bread recipe, p. 229) and serve with Sesame-free Hummus, p. 220 or Parsley Pesto, p. 221 (contains cashews so may not be allowed at school)

Mid-morning snack	Lunch	Afternoon snack
Day 5 'Friday is treat day'		
Choose from: Pear Muffin, p. 249; banana; or Papaya Rice Paper Rolls, p. 230 Water bottle (filtered water)	Design Your Own Sandwich, p. 228 or wheat-free sandwich with Banana Carob Spread, p. 220	New Anzac Cookies, p. 250 or vanilla soy yoghurt (no 160b/annatto) with Banana Carob Spread, p. 220 or papaya and chopped canned pear Pack a spoon and freezer block

(*You can use dinner leftovers for lunch, and most of the recipes in Chapter 18 are suitable. Just be sure to adjust the portions and cut up foods into smaller bite-sizes to suit your child's age and feeding ability.)

The Eczema Diet: Stage 1

Your child's skin should show signs of improvement within two to four weeks. And after strictly following the diet and supplement routine for two months your child's skin condition should be mostly or completely clear. If this does not occur, suspect they are eating something they are sensitive to (for example rice or spelt, which feature heavily in the diet).

The Eczema Diet: Stage 2

As eczema symptoms disappear, food variety is expanded to Stage 2. I recommend waiting until your child's eczema completely disappears before reintroducing foods into the diet in Stage 2. However, if your child is unhappy and wants to eat a greater range of foods, then increase variety sooner rather than later. Stage 2 information can be found in Chapter 17, 'Stage 2: Expanding the diet'.

General recommendations

- Make your child as comfortable as possible and use their prescribed medicated creams if desired.
- Photocopy the 'Eczema-safe shopping guide: Stage 1' pp. 260–261 so you can take it with you when you go grocery shopping.
- If desired, keep a copy of the table on p. 157, 'How many serves per day for children', on the fridge.
- If desired, you can photocopy the menus and have them on the fridge and/or use the blank diet diary at the back of the book to record what your child is eating. This can help you identify problematic foods (and beneficial meals) so you can tailor the program to suit your child.
- Before starting the program, read Chapter 12, 'Getting started'.
- It's highly recommended that the whole family enjoy the eczema-safe recipes. When families share eczema-safe meals it can help a child with eczema to feel 'normal' and compliance is more likely.

Chapter 15

Party food guide + lolly bags

While party food generally causes itchy skin and a worsening of symptoms, it's possible to have an eczema-safe birthday party and other special occasions such as Christmas. The party food guide given on p. 183 is suitable for adults and children over the age of one. These items are suggestions to choose from — you don't need to serve all of the listed items. Ensure you choose items to suit the partygoers' ages, allergies and feeding abilities. For example, a one-year-old child may not be able to eat hard foods such as toffee and if someone is allergic to nuts (e.g. peanuts) then it's best to avoid serving cashew-containing foods.

Lolly bags

Children usually like to have take-home bags of sweets given to them at the end of a party. If you choose to have them, the items marked with an asterisk* in the table on p. 183 may be suitable lolly bag treats, depending on the age and feeding ability of the children attending the party. Non-food additions to the lolly bag can include kids bracelets, cheap jewellery, homemade beaded items, balloons, whistles, mini plastic dinosaurs and other small figurines from a discount shop.

Below are some ideas for what to include in your eczema-safe lolly bags.

Lolly bag 1
- caramels (plain, no additives or chocolate)
- white marshmallows
- plastic bracelet or figurine
- balloon
- whistle or mini bubble blower (if not sensitive to dishwashing liquid)

Lolly bag 2

- Eczema-safe cupcake with plain icing, wrapped in clear or coloured cellophane and tied with a colourful ribbon (Birthday Cake recipe, p. 246)
- stickers

Lolly bag 3

- white marshmallows
- honeycomb
- balloon
- stickers

The truth about sugar

Although unhealthy sugar-rich and fried foods are listed as eczema-safe in this chapter, I strongly recommend avoiding having these foods on a daily or regular basis. Most of these eczema-safe party foods and drinks are considered unhealthy as they take more nutrients to process than they supply, so they deplete the body of valuable nutrients needed for healthy skin. Furthermore, sugary foods increase acid in the body, so they may exacerbate the itch.

To help counteract the negative effects from eating sugar-rich or fried foods, drink a glass of highly alkalising juice such as Tarzan Juice (p. 222) or Healthy Skin Juice (p. 222), or eat Alkaline Bomb Salad (p. 233) or add mung bean sprouts to your next meal to help restore your acid–alkaline balance.

Occasional treats

If you would like to treat yourself or your child occasionally, give yourself strict guidelines. If you stick within these guidelines it should not affect your results (or might only delay them slightly). Firstly, only have treats from the list of 'eczema-safe' treats in this chapter. Secondly, set yourself/your child a *specific day and time* when you can enjoy a treat. For example, 'treat day is Sunday', when you can have maple syrup on pancakes for breakfast (using eczema-safe ingredients) and later have a couple of marshmallows after lunch or dinner and Choco Milk after dinner or as a morning snack. Other examples include 'iceblock day is Friday' (only consume plain lemonade iceblocks/popsicles/ice lollies), or for the adults: 'I can drink alcohol at birthday parties and weddings' (two glasses or less of eczema-safe alcohol per fortnight, see table below). If you are craving sweet foods or alcohol, find out what your cravings might indicate on p. 77, 'Sugar cravings'.

Eczema-safe party foods	Eczema-safe home-prepared items
lemonade, bottled (no colours, unpreserved) natural mineral water (no flavours or colour)	jug of filtered water, chilled
soda water	Birthday Cake, p. 246
lemonade iceblocks/popsicles/ice lollies, plain (no colours or preservatives)	cupcakes* (Birthday Cake recipe, p. 246)
potato crisps/chips/fries (plain salted, no colour, no flavour enhancer or additives)	Baked Banana Chips, p. 218
mini packets of plain potato crisps*	carrot and celery sticks served with Parsley Pesto, p. 221 (contains cashews) or Sesame-free Hummus, p. 220
rice crackers (plain, salted, no flavour enhancer or additives, no corn/maize)	Potato Wedges, p. 218 (need to be cooked just before serving and served warm)
green soy beans/edamame (available from sushi restaurants)	New Anzac Biscuits, p. 250
plain caramels* (no number additives)	Papaya Rice Paper Rolls, p. 230
plain toffee* (no number additives)	spelt chips (use Spelt Lavash Bread recipe, p. 229), served with Sesame-free Hummus, p. 220
white marshmallows*	
honeycomb	
Adults only	
gin	decaffeinated coffee (with soy milk)
tonic water, bottled (no preservatives)	unsalted cashews, raw
vodka and soda	
whisky and soda	

* May be suitable treats to place in lolly bags.

Chapter 16
Adult/family menu

The adult menu begins with a 3-day Alkalising Cleanse, where you eat predominantly alkalising ingredients to enhance liver detoxification of chemicals and cleanse the digestive tract. This food-based cleanse is optional and is a great way to kick-start your healthy skin program if you choose to follow it. There is a 14-day meal plan which can be repeated or you can adapt the menus to suit your preferences. If you are feeding your family, the meals listed in the adult menus can be enjoyed by everyone from day 4 onwards.

3-day Alkalising Cleanse

The 3-day Alkalising Cleanse is a highly nutritious and gentle food-based cleanse that is gluten-free, low in natural chemicals and contains no artificial chemicals. The three-day cleanse is not suitable for children, pregnant or breastfeeding women, or anyone who has a medical condition requiring medical drugs.

If you are used to consuming caffeine and sugar, or if you have candidiasis, you might feel tired during the cleanse and might experience headaches as you go through caffeine, sugar and/or chemical withdrawals. Candida die-off can also cause these symptoms. If you feel tired it's advisable to rest, relax and refrain from exercise, and drink plenty of filtered water.

Recipes for the 3-day Alkalising Cleanse
- Therapeutic Broth, p. 226
- Alkaline Vegie Broth, p. 225 (alternative broth for vegetarians and vegans)
- New Potato and Leek Soup, p. 234
- Chickpea Casserole, p. 242
- Tarzan Juice, p. 222

During the cleanse

- Enhance Phase 2 liver detoxification by cooking with fresh garlic and eat either cabbage or brussels sprouts daily (these are included in the recipes).
- Drink filtered water (five to eight glasses daily).
- Eat raw vegies daily: celery, mung bean sprouts, spring onions (scallions), iceberg lettuce (no other raw vegies during the cleanse).
- Herbs to choose from are chives and parsley.
- You can eat the following steamed vegies: cabbage, green beans, brussels sprouts, white potato (potatoes to avoid are listed on p. 260 in the shopping guide), and eat choko (chayote) if desired (though choko is not essential).
- Don't go hungry: eat as much soup, casserole and/or raw vegies as you like and drink plenty of Tarzan Juice (at least two glasses).
- It's important to rest and not go out socialising during the cleanse as you need to avoid all other foods and drinks for three days.

Main menu recipe list

After completing the 3-day Alkalising Cleanse, if you choose to do it, you can select from the following list a range of meals each day. Alternatively, you can refer to the handy menus starting on p. 190.

Breakfast selection

(The first three recipes are the preferred choices.)

- Surprise Porridge, p. 215
- Omega Muesli, p. 214
- Quinoa Porridge, p. 216
- Healthy Skin Smoothie, p. 223
- Spelt Pancakes, p. 247
- Buckwheat Crepes, p. 248
- spelt sourdough toast or gluten-free bread with Banana Carob Spread, p. 220

- Spelt Lavash Bread, p. 229
- Pear Muffins, p. 249
- puffed brown rice, plain puffed rice cereal

Drink selection

- filtered water
- Tarzan Juice, p. 222
- Healthy Skin Juice, p. 222
- Therapeutic Broth, p. 226
- Alkaline Vegie Broth, p. 225 (alternative broth for vegetarians and vegans)
- Healthy Skin Smoothie, p. 223

Snack selection

- carrot and celery sticks with Sesame-free Hummus, p. 220
- Alkaline Bomb Salad, p. 233
- The Wishing Plate, p. 217
- Papaya Rice Paper Rolls, p. 230
- sliced papaya, peeled pear, banana
- Eczema-safe Fruit Salad, p. 217
- Pear Muffins, p. 249
- Baked Banana Chips, p. 218
- plain rice crackers (no additives) with Bean Dip, p. 219
- wholegrain rye crispbread with Parsley Pesto, p. 221
- wholegrain rice cakes with Banana Carob Spread, p. 220
- Potato Wedges, p. 218 (homemade)
- Banana Icy Poles, p. 245
- Stewed Pear, p. 248

Lunch and dinner selection

- New Potato and Leek Soup, p. 234
- Papaya Rice Paper Rolls, p. 230
- Design Your Own Sandwich, p. 228

- Roasted Sweet Potato Salad, p. 233
- Roasted Potato Stack, p. 232
- Sunshine Soup, p. 235
- Baked Fish with Mash, p. 237
- Easy Roast Chicken, p. 240 with Eczema-safe Gravy, p. 240
- Country Chicken Soup, p. 236
- Cinnamon Chicken, p. 241
- Chickpea Casserole, p. 242
- Chickpea Rice, p. 231
- Alkaline Bomb Salad, p. 233 with optional chicken, fish or lamb
- Sticks and Stones (fish or chicken on skewers), p. 238
- My Favourite Lamb Cutlets, p. 243
- Pasta, p. 244

DIY suggestions

I encourage you to experiment with the eczema-safe ingredients and create your own meals, for example:

- lean lamb/chicken/fish/veal with green beans, brussels sprouts and Smashed Potato, p. 239
- lean lamb/chicken/fish/veal/beans with roasted carrots and Potato Wedges, p. 218
- grilled chicken served with Alkaline Bomb Salad, p. 233
- vegetarians and vegans: plain tofu with kidney beans, quinoa and diced carrots
- chicken casserole with potatoes, sweet potato, carrots, leeks and celery (modify the Chickpea Casserole recipe, p. 242).

Must you eat meat?

Please note it is not necessary to eat red meat, fish or chicken during the Eczema Diet. Recipes containing meat are in the menu mainly for variety (and they supply protein and iron). Please choose vegetarian soups and eat beans if preferred.

Vegetarians and vegans

Eczema-safe vegetarian protein sources are chickpeas (garbanzo beans), green beans, raw cashews (if no nut allergy), tofu, lentils, kidney beans and other beans (not broad beans). Most of the Eczema Diet recipes can be converted so they are suitable for vegetarians and vegans, with the exception of Easy Roast Chicken, Baked Fish with Mash and Therapeutic Broth (Alkaline Vegie Broth, p. 225, is a suitable broth alternative). If a dinner recipe contains animal product and it cannot be converted to a vegetarian or vegan meal, then an option marked with 'V&Vn' will be given or there will be soup options. Many of the recipes in the menus are already suitable for vegetarians and vegans (such as breakfasts and snacks) and these are not marked with 'V&Vn'.

Avoid these: tempeh, vegan/vegetarian patties and sausages, and other meat substitutes as they can contain additives, soy sauce and/or natural flavourings and herbs so they are not eczema-safe.

Gluten intolerance

If you cannot eat gluten, there are gluten-free meal suggestions within the menus and these are marked with 'GF' in the recipes. The 3-day Alkalising Cleanse is gluten-free.

Rate your eczema

At the bottom of the menus where it says 'Rate your eczema' you have the option to make notes about your skin as you progress through the diet. If you suspect an adverse reaction to a particular food or an environmental exposure, write it down on the lines provided. You can also rate your eczema from 1 to 10: a score of 1 (shown as 1/10) means your eczema is at its worst and covering a large part of your body; a score of 10/10 would indicate that your eczema is no longer present. Before beginning the program, you may also like to take photos of your eczema so you can document your skin condition before and after.

The menus

The following menus are guides only: you'll need to adjust them to suit your allergies and appetite. These symbols ★ ● P ♦ ✳ appear at the top of each column in the menus as a reminder to have some vegies, fruit, wholegrains, protein or liquids at that particular meal break. You don't have to strictly follow these suggestions, but if it becomes a habit for you to think 'Lunch time is when I serve wholegrains', or 'I'll serve protein with dinner', it will be easier to have a balanced diet.

The following menus are free of wheat, dairy, nuts and eggs, and contain alkalising foods and drinks. The menus can be made vegetarian or vegan with a few minor changes (read vegetarian and vegan information, opposite), and choose gluten-free ingredients if you are gluten intolerant. You'll see there is a 'treat day' every seventh day and every food break there are several meal choices (also refer to the lists in this chapter and the 'Eczema-safe shopping guide: Stage 1', pp. 260–261).

When following the meal plan, you can eat more or less food depending on your appetite and health requirements. For example, if you are very thin or frail you may need to add some baked goods such as Pear Muffins into your daily routine or eat Omega Muesli for dessert. Do not go hungry. This is not a weight-loss program although weight loss may be experienced if you are accustomed to eating high-fat or sugar-rich processed foods.

Rate your eczema

Rate your eczema the day before you start the program.
Day 0: __/ __/ ____   Skin condition: ___/10

Cleanse day 1

Breakfast ◆ ★	Morning snack ★	Lunch ★ P ☀
Supplements with filtered water or Tarzan Juice, p. 222 Baked potatoes (no oil) with celery and mung bean sprouts; optional: ½ cup warm broth	Choose from: salad: iceberg lettuce, celery, mung bean sprouts, spring onion (scallions); or steamed baby potatoes and green beans topped with chopped chives Tarzan Juice, p. 222 or filtered water	New Potato and Leek Soup, p. 234 Filtered water

Afternoon snack ★	Dinner P ★	Rate your eczema: /10
Choose from: salad: iceberg lettuce, celery, mung bean sprouts, spring onion (scallions); or steamed baby potatoes and green beans topped with chopped chives Tarzan Juice, p. 222 or filtered water	Chickpea Casserole, p. 242 (1–2 serves, do not go hungry) Filtered water	Notes

Cleanse day 2

Breakfast ◆ ★	Morning snack ★	Lunch ★ P ✳
Supplements with filtered water or Tarzan Juice, p. 222 Choose from: baked potato (no oil) with celery and mung bean sprouts; or New Potato and Leek Soup, p. 234	Choose from: salad: iceberg lettuce, celery, mung bean sprouts, spring onion (scallions); or steamed baby potatoes and green beans topped with chopped chives Tarzan Juice, p. 222 or filtered water	New Potato and Leek Soup, p. 234 Filtered water

Afternoon snack ★	Dinner P ★	Rate your eczema: /10
Choose from: salad: iceberg lettuce, celery, mung bean sprouts, spring onion (scallions); or steamed baby potatoes and green beans topped with chopped chives Tarzan Juice, p. 222 or filtered water	Chickpea Casserole, p. 242 (1–2 serves, do not go hungry) Filtered water	Notes

Cleanse day 3

Breakfast ◆ ★	Morning snack ★	Lunch ★ P ✳
Supplements with filtered water or Tarzan Juice, p. 222 Choose from: baked potato (no oil) with celery and mung bean sprouts; or New Potato and Leek Soup, p. 234	Choose from: salad: iceberg lettuce, celery, mung bean sprouts, spring onion (scallions); or steamed baby potatoes and green beans topped with chopped chives Tarzan Juice, p. 222 or filtered water	New Potato and Leek Soup, p. 234 Filtered water

Afternoon snack ★	Dinner P ★	Rate your eczema: /10
Choose from: salad: iceberg lettuce, celery, mung bean sprouts, spring onion (scallions); or steamed baby potatoes and green beans topped with chopped chives Tarzan Juice, p. 222 or filtered water	Chickpea Casserole, p. 242 (1–2 serves, do not go hungry) Filtered water (Soak oats or quinoa for tomorrow's breakfast, see day 4, opposite)	Notes

Day 4

Breakfast ◐ ★

Supplements with filtered water or Healthy Skin Juice, p. 222

Choose from: Omega Muesli, p. 214; Surprise Porridge, p. 215; Quinoa Porridge, p. 216; or Healthy Skin Smoothie, p. 223

(Make Therapeutic Broth if you have run out, p. 226)

Morning snack 🍎

Choose from: papaya, banana or peeled pear; Eczema-safe Fruit Salad, p. 217; or Healthy Skin Smoothie, p. 223

Filtered water and/or Healthy Skin Juice, p. 222

Lunch ★ P ☀

Choose from: Design Your Own Sandwich, p. 228; Papaya Rice Paper Rolls, p. 230; Roasted Sweet Potato Salad, p. 233; or Roasted Potato Stack, p. 232 (all have GF options)

Filtered water

Afternoon snack ★

Choose from: carrot and celery sticks with Sesame-free Hummus, p. 220 and brown rice crackers; or Alkaline Bomb Salad, p. 233

Filtered water or Healthy Skin Juice, p. 222

Dinner P ★

Choose from: Baked Fish with Mush, p. 237, or soup of choice, pp. 234–236

Rate your eczema: /10

Notes

Day 5

Breakfast ♦ ★

Supplements with filtered water or Tarzan Juice, p. 222

Choose from: Omega Muesli, p. 214; Surprise Porridge, p. 215; Quinoa Porridge, p. 216; or Healthy Skin Smoothie, p. 223

Morning snack 🍎

Choose from: papaya, banana or peeled pear; Eczema-safe Fruit Salad, p. 217; or Healthy Skin Smoothie, p. 223

Filtered water and/or Healthy Skin Juice, p. 222

Lunch ★ P ✳

Choose from: Design Your Own Sandwich, p. 228; Papaya Rice Paper Rolls, p. 230; Roasted Sweet Potato Salad, p. 233; or Roasted Potato Stack, p. 232 (all have GF options)

Filtered water

Afternoon snack ★

Choose from: carrot and celery sticks with Sesame-free Hummus, p. 220 and brown rice crackers; or Alkaline Bomb Salad, p. 233

Filtered water or Tarzan Juice, p. 222

Dinner P ★

Choose from: Cinnamon Chicken, p. 241; or soup of choice, pp. 234–236

Rate your eczema: /10

Notes

Day 6

Breakfast ♦ ★

Supplements with filtered water or Healthy Skin Juice, p. 222

Choose from: Omega Muesli, p. 214; Surprise Porridge, p. 215; Quinoa Porridge, p. 216; or Healthy Skin Smoothie, p. 223

Morning snack 🍎

Choose from: papaya, banana or peeled pear; Eczema-safe Fruit Salad, p. 217; or Healthy Skin Smoothie, p. 223

Filtered water and/or Healthy Skin Juice, p. 222

Lunch ☀

Choose from: Design Your Own Sandwich, p. 228; Papaya Rice Paper Rolls, p. 230; Roasted Sweet Potato Salad, p. 233; or Roasted Potato Stack, p. 232 (all have GF options)

Filtered water

Afternoon snack ★

Choose from: carrot and celery sticks with Sesame-free Hummus, p. 220 and brown rice crackers; or Alkaline Bomb Salad, p. 233

Filtered water or Healthy Skin Juice, p. 222

Dinner P ★

Choose from: Sticks and Stones, p. 238 (skewers); or soup of choice, pp. 234–236 (needs 3 cups of broth, p. 226)

Rate your eczema: /10

Notes

Day 7 (Treat Day)

Breakfast ◆ ★	Morning snack ●	Lunch ✳
Supplements with filtered water or Tarzan Juice, p. 222 Choose from: Omega Muesli, p. 214; Spelt Pancakes, p. 247; Buckwheat Crepes, p. 248; or Healthy Skin Smoothie, p. 223	Choose from: Banana Icy Pole, p. 245, papaya or peeled pear; Eczema-safe Fruit Salad, p. 217; or Healthy Skin Smoothie, p. 223 Filtered water and/or Healthy Skin Juice, p. 222	Choose from: Spelt Lavash Bread, p. 229 with salad or Banana Carob Spread, p. 220; Design Your Own Sandwich, p. 228; Papaya Rice Paper Rolls, p. 230; or Roasted Potato Stack, p. 232 (all have GF options) Filtered water

Afternoon snack ★	Dinner P ★	Rate your eczema: /10
Choose from: carrot and celery sticks with Sesame-free Hummus, p. 220 and brown rice crackers; Alkaline Bomb Salad, p. 233; or Potato Wedges, p. 218 and Sesame-free Hummus, p. 220 Filtered water or Tarzan Juice, p. 222	Choose from: Easy Roast Chicken, p. 240; or soup of choice, pp. 234–236; or Chickpea Rice, p. 231 (V&Vn) Optional dessert: Choco Milk, p. 245; Banana Icy Poles, p. 245; or Baked Banana Chips, p. 218	**Notes**

Day 8

Breakfast ● ★

Supplements with filtered water or Healthy Skin Juice, p. 222

Choose from: Omega Muesli, p. 214; Surprise Porridge, p. 215; Quinoa Porridge, p. 216; or Healthy Skin Smoothie, p. 223

(Make Therapeutic Broth if you have run out, p. 226)

Morning snack ●

Choose from: papaya, banana or peeled pear; Eczema-safe Fruit Salad, p. 217; or Healthy Skin Smoothie, p. 223

Filtered water and/or Healthy Skin Juice, p. 222

Lunch ●

Choose from: Design Your Own Sandwich, p. 228; Papaya Rice Paper Rolls, p. 230; Roasted Sweet Potato Salad, p. 233; or Roasted Potato Stack, p. 232 (all have GF options)

Filtered water

Afternoon snack ★

Choose from: carrot and celery sticks with Sesame-free Hummus, p. 220 and brown rice crackers; or Alkaline Bomb Salad, p. 233

Filtered water or Healthy Skin Juice, p. 222

Dinner P ★

Choose from: Chickpea Rice, p. 231 (with leftover roast chicken); or soup of choice, pp. 234–236

Rate your eczema: /10

Notes

Day 9

Breakfast ◆ ★

Supplements with filtered water or Tarzan Juice, p. 222

Choose from: Omega Muesli, p. 214; Surprise Porridge, p. 215; Quinoa Porridge, p. 216; or Healthy Skin Smoothie, p. 223

Morning snack 🍎

Choose from: papaya, banana or peeled pear; Eczema-safe Fruit Salad, p. 217; or Healthy Skin Smoothie, p. 223

Filtered water and/or Healthy Skin Juice, p. 222

Lunch ❋

Choose from: Design Your Own Sandwich, p. 228; Papaya Rice Paper Rolls, p. 230; Roasted Sweet Potato Salad, p. 233; or Roasted Potato Stack, p. 232 (all have GF options)

Filtered water

Afternoon snack ★

Choose from: carrot and celery sticks with Sesame-free Hummus, p. 220 and brown rice crackers; or Alkaline Bomb Salad, p. 233

Filtered water or Tarzan Juice, p. 222

Dinner P ★

Choose from: Sunshine Soup, p. 235; or soup of choice, pp. 234–236

Rate your eczema: /10

Notes

Day 10

Breakfast ◆ ★

Supplements with filtered water or Healthy Skin Juice, p. 222

Choose from: Omega Muesli, p. 214; Surprise Porridge, p. 215; Quinoa Porridge, p. 216; or Healthy Skin Smoothie, p. 223

Morning snack 🍎

Choose from: papaya, banana or peeled pear; Eczema-safe Fruit Salad, p. 217; or Healthy Skin Smoothie, p. 223

Filtered water and/or Healthy Skin Juice, p. 222

Lunch ☀

Choose from: Design Your Own Sandwich, p. 228; Papaya Rice Paper Rolls, p. 230; Roasted Sweet Potato Salad, p. 233; or Roasted Potato Stack, p. 232 (all have GF options)

Filtered water

Afternoon snack ★

Choose from: carrot and celery sticks with Sesame-free Hummus, p. 220 and brown rice crackers; or Alkaline Bomb Salad, p. 233

Filtered water or Healthy Skin Juice, p. 222

Dinner P ★

Choose from: Chickpea Casserole, p. 242; Papaya Rice Paper Rolls, p. 230 (served with rice or salad); or soup of choice, pp. 234–236

Rate your eczema: /10

Notes

Day 11

Breakfast ◆ ★	Morning snack 🍎	Lunch ✳
Supplements with filtered water or Healthy Skin Juice, p. 222	Choose from: papaya, banana or peeled pear; Eczema-safe Fruit Salad, p. 217; or Healthy Skin Smoothie, p. 223	Choose from: Design Your Own Sandwich, p. 228; Papaya Rice Paper Rolls, p. 230; Roasted Sweet Potato Salad, p. 233; or Roasted Potato Stack, p. 232 (all have GF options)
Choose from: Omega Muesli, p. 214; Surprise Porridge, p. 215; Quinoa Porridge, p. 216; or Healthy Skin Smoothie, p. 223	Filtered water and/or Healthy Skin Juice, p. 222	Filtered water

Afternoon snack ★	Dinner P ★	Rate your eczema: /10
Choose from: carrot and celery sticks with Sesame-free Hummus, p. 220 and brown rice crackers; or Alkaline Bomb Salad, p. 233	Choose from: Pasta, p. 244; or soup of choice, pp. 234–236	**Notes**
Filtered water or Healthy Skin Juice, p. 222		

Day 12

Breakfast ♦ ★

Supplements with filtered water or Healthy Skin Juice, p. 222

Choose from: Omega Muesli, p. 214; Surprise Porridge, p. 215; Quinoa Porridge, p. 216; or Healthy Skin Smoothie, p. 223

(Make Therapeutic Broth if you have run out, p. 226)

Morning snack 🍎

Choose from: papaya, banana or peeled pear; Eczema-safe Fruit Salad, p. 217; or Healthy Skin Smoothie, p. 223

Filtered water and/or Healthy Skin Juice, p. 222

Lunch ☀

Choose from: Design Your Own Sandwich, p. 228; Papaya Rice Paper Rolls, p. 230; Roasted Sweet Potato Salad, p. 233; or Roasted Potato Stack, p. 232 (all have GF options)

Filtered water

Afternoon snack ★

Choose from: carrot and celery sticks with Sesame-free Hummus, p. 220 and brown rice crackers; or Alkaline Bomb Salad, p. 233

Filtered water or Healthy Skin Juice, p. 222

Dinner P ★

Choose from: My Favourite Lamb Cutlets, p. 243; or soup of choice, pp. 234–236

Dessert: papaya (rich in vitamin C to help iron absorption)

Rate your eczema: /10

Notes

Day 13

Breakfast ◊ ★

Supplements with filtered water or Tarzan Juice, p. 222

Choose from: Omega Muesli, p. 214; Surprise Porridge, p. 215; Quinoa Porridge, p. 216; or Healthy Skin Smoothie, p. 223

Morning snack ●

Choose from: papaya, banana or peeled pear; Eczema-safe Fruit Salad, p. 217; or Healthy Skin Smoothie, p. 223

Filtered water and/or Healthy Skin Juice, p. 222

Lunch ☀

Choose from: Design Your Own Sandwich, p. 228; Papaya Rice Paper Rolls, p. 230; Roasted Sweet Potato Salad, p. 233; or Roasted Potato Stack, p. 232 (all have GF options)

Filtered water

Afternoon snack ★

Choose from: carrot and celery sticks with Sesame-free Hummus, p. 220 and brown rice crackers; or Alkaline Bomb Salad, p. 233

Filtered water or Tarzan Juice, p. 222

Dinner P ★

Choose from: Baked Fish with Mash, p. 237 (use eczema-safe white fish, p. 72); or soup of choice, pp. 234–236

Rate your eczema: /10

Notes

Day 14 (Treat day)

Breakfast ◐ ★

Supplements with filtered water or Healthy Skin Juice, p. 222

Choose from: Omega Muesli, p. 214; Spelt Pancakes, p. 247; Buckwheat Crepes, p. 248; or Healthy Skin Smoothie, p. 223

Morning snack 🍎

Choose from: Baked Banana Chips, p. 218; papaya, banana or peeled pear; Eczema-safe Fruit Salad, p. 217; or Healthy Skin Smoothie, p. 223

Filtered water and/or Healthy Skin Juice, p. 222

Lunch ✳

Choose from: Spelt Lavash Bread, p. 229 with salad or Banana Carob Spread, p. 220; Design Your Own Sandwich, p. 228; Papaya Rice Paper Rolls, p. 230; or Roasted Potato Stack, p. 232 (all have GF options)

Filtered water

Afternoon snack ★

Choose from: carrot and celery sticks with Sesame-free Hummus, p. 220 and brown rice crackers; Alkaline Bomb Salad, p. 233; or Potato Wedges, p. 218 and Sesame-free Hummus, p. 220

Filtered water or Healthy Skin Juice, p. 222

Dinner P ★

Choose from: Easy Roast Chicken, p. 240; or soup of choice (V&Vn), pp. 234–236

Optional dessert: Choco Milk, p. 245; Banana Icy Poles, p. 245; or Baked Banana Chips, p. 218

Rate your eczema: /10

Notes

Continue with the Eczema Diet by repeating this two-week program for eight weeks, or by designing your own program using the eczema-safe ingredients and recipes. For best results take the eczema supplements during the program and for a minimum of twelve weeks.

Recommendations

Before beginning the Eczema Diet read Chapter 12, 'Getting started'.

Chapter 17

Stage 2: Expanding the diet

Stage 2 is the second part of the Eczema Diet where you can eat other types of foods, along with the Stage 1 ingredients. This is an important step to increase the variety of foods in your diet and this stage can also help you identify food sensitivities. Particular foods have been selected for Stage 2 because they add extra nutrients and flavours to the diet (and I thought you might like them), plus they meet *all* of the following criteria:

- they have health properties, such as being alkalising or rich in flavonoids
- they contain 'medium' or 'high' salicylates; not 'very high' (with the exception of apple cider vinegar, which is also highly alkalising)

When is it a good time to begin Stage 2 of the Eczema Diet?

It's up to you when you begin Stage 2. On saying this, rushing into Stage 2 prematurely can set you back and may affect your results. The following are basic guidelines for moving on to Stage 2:

1. You need your eczema to be visibly improving and your skin holding moisture better. It is a good sign if you can start using a lighter moisturiser and your skin is in a healing phase (not flared up and showing signs of healing).

2. You need your eczema to be *consistently* improving. If you are still having random, unexplained flare-ups you need to do some additional investigation to identify what you are reacting to (and then stop exposing yourself to it).

3. You need to be happy with your results before moving onto Stage 2.

I recommend waiting until your eczema has completely healed before moving onto Stage 2. The only reason to move ahead to Stage 2 at a faster pace would be if you had to increase the range of foods in your diet due to boredom or fussy eating habits and you were happy to risk slowing down your results (on saying this, you may find Stage 2 foods don't cause any adverse reactions so you can happily expand your diet).

When introducing a new food, such as blueberries, it's best to begin with small amounts only, as the over-consumption of one or two Stage 2 foods may cause flare-ups (and dishearten you!). If you are quite sensitive, you may like to begin by eating your favourite Stage 2 ingredients in small portions once a week and slowly build up to two or more times a week.

Stage 2 vegetables

All vegetables are alkalising so it's important to expand your range as soon as possible. Try one new food every three days and note any adverse reactions in your diet diary. If an adverse reaction occurs, discontinue use and re-test the food in two months' time, if desired. Add these medium salicylate vegetables into your diet:

- asparagus
- bok choy (pak choy)
- snow pea (mangetout)
- snow pea (mangetout) sprouts
- endive
- chicory
- mint
- basil (in moderation)
- coriander (cilantro)
- baby (pattypan) squash
- turnip
- yam
- fresh/frozen green peas (contains natural MSG)

Organic tomato sauce

Tomato is an important part of Stage 2 as it's rich in skin-protective lycopene. The most powerful antioxidant of all the carotenoids, lycopene can reduce the risk of skin cancer and prostate cancer, and if consumed regularly, it has a mild protective effect against sunburn. Cooked tomato contains more lycopene than raw. However, tomato is traditionally problematic for eczema sufferers as it's rich in natural MSG, which gives tomato products their lovely flavour. Raw tomato may be the most problematic so it's best to eat cooked tomato and *only in moderation.*

Plain organic tomato sauce has been chosen for Stage 2 as it is pleasant for all ages to consume (especially children) and it should have no artificial additives. It is an *optional* addition to your diet if you miss using sauce. Begin with 1 teaspoon once or twice a week (a maximum of 1 teaspoon for children and 2 teaspoons for adults, up to three times a week). If you have an adverse reaction to tomato sauce, discontinue use. Alternatively, you can eat a slice of papaya daily to ensure you consume lycopene in the diet (this is most important).

Onions

White and red onions are rich in the flavonoid quercetin, so onions can make a nutritious addition to your diet. Onions are high in salicylates so try the other Stage 2 vegetables first and if no adverse reactions occur, you may like to test onions (eating onions in the diet is optional). Discontinue use if you have an adverse reaction to them.

All other vegetables, such as spinach (**SS, M, A**) and broccoli (**SS, M, A**), are very high in salicylates and other natural chemicals so do not eat them just yet. You can expand your vegetable range further once Stage 2 vegetables have passed the test.

Stage 2 fruits

Stage 2 fruits contain medium salicylates and they have been chosen as they are highly nutritious. Note that blueberries and lemons are high in salicylates (lemon also contains lots of amines), but they have been chosen for Stage 2 because of their rich antioxidant content and for lemon's strong alkalising effect; and watermelon contains lycopene. Add these salicylate fruits into your diet (one every three days, if desired):

- golden delicious apples and red delicious (other varieties are high in salicylates)
- watermelon
- blueberries (SS)(AA)
- lemon or lime (SS)(AA)

How to test lemon

First test the other fruits such as red delicious apples, watermelon and blueberries. If they all pass the test (and your eczema does not return) then consume 1 teaspoon of lemon juice each day for one to three days. If no reaction occurs, try the Flaxseed Lemon Drink, p. 223. Lemon is useful for flavouring fish and pasta recipes and the Flaxseed Lemon Drink is fantastic for the skin (if you don't have an adverse reaction to the lemon). If an adverse reaction occurs, note it in your diet diary, discontinue use and re-test lemon in one to two months' time if desired.

Stage 2 spices

Spices can offer you an impressive range of flavonoids, antioxidants and delicious flavours that make a diet rich and interesting. Cinnamon and cumin are two of the most valuable spices for eczema sufferers. If these ones don't cause flare-ups you can try other spices such as whole nutmeg (grated onto porridge), basil and mixed herbs in casseroles or dried mint flakes on lamb. One range of spices you may have ongoing problems with is curry powder as it is incredibly rich in salicylates so don't try curry just yet. Cinnamon and cumin contain high salicylates but they can be used in small amounts.

Cinnamon

Cinnamon plays a starring role in Stage 2 because this delicious spice contains cinnamaldehyde which lowers blood glucose level and slows the absorption of carbohydrates in the intestines.[1] To test it, add a sprinkling of cinnamon to Omega Muesli, p. 214, Quinoa Porridge, p.216 or Surprise Porridge, p. 215 and then see if there are any adverse reactions in the three days that follow. If an adverse reaction occurs, note it in your diet diary, discontinue use and re-test cinnamon in one to two months' time. (Continue taking a chromium supplement as chromium also improves blood glucose tolerance.)

If there is no adverse reaction, you can add it to foods such as Cinnamon Chicken, p. 241 or sprinkle it onto potatoes before baking to help lower your blood insulin level (which can spike after eating potato and carbohydrate-rich grains). If you are allergic to cinnamon avoid it and test nutmeg instead as it also helps with blood sugar control. Buy whole nutmeg and finely grate it onto your breakfast cereals or use it whenever you use rice milk.

Ground cumin

Cumin can decrease blood sugar and it contains antioxidants which are beneficial for the heart. It makes recipes such as hummus, casseroles and meat dishes taste delicious. Add a sprinkling of ground cumin to Sesame-free Hummus, p. 220 and if no adverse reaction occurs add it to Chickpea Casserole, p. 242 or sprinkle it onto Easy Roast Chicken, p. 240.

Other Stage 2 additions

Important note: Below are a range of handy *alkalising* foods you might like to reintroduce into your diet at this stage. These three ingredients may cause adverse reactions and it is not essential to add these to your diet.

Butter (pure organic)

This Stage 2 addition is optional and it's introduced during Stage 2 for your convenience — do not use butter if you have an allergy to dairy products. Butter was chosen because pure organic butter contains no additives and it's slightly alkalising when unheated. It's the least reactive of all the dairy products so it may be well tolerated if you don't have an allergy to dairy products. Do not use butter for cooking as the smoking point is too low and if an adverse reaction occurs, note it in your diet diary, discontinue use and, if desired, re-test dairy products in two months' time. As this product is rich in saturated fats, it's essential to keep butter use to a minimum.

Apple cider vinegar

Vinegar can be handy for making delicious salad dressings and this one has health benefits too. While most vinegars are strongly acid-forming and unsuitable for eczema sufferers, apple cider vinegar is highly alkalising and it can be beneficial for eczema. There is a catch, however. Apple cider vinegar is rich in natural chemicals including sulfites, salicylates and moderate amines, so it may cause your eczema to return, especially if you are sensitive to sulfites (if you have sulfite allergy do not test apple cider vinegar).

If you do not have sulfite sensitivity, test apple cider vinegar in the delicious salad dressing recipe Omega Salad Dressing, p. 219. Wait up to three days to see if there is an adverse reaction. If an adverse reaction occurs, note it in your diet diary and discontinue use. Alternatively, once this ingredient has passed the test, you can use the dressing on salads such as Alkaline Bomb Salad, p. 233 and Roasted Sweet Potato Salad, p. 233. Apple cider vinegar has potent antibacterial and preserving qualities so you can use a splash of apple cider vinegar in water to wash vegetables and sprouts.

Chlorophyll

Chlorophyll is the green pigment in plants, and it's also a green alkalising supplement that assists with digestion and detoxification. Chlorella is often used as it's a rich source of chlorophyll. The supplement is available in liquid and tablet form, however the liquid varieties usually have added preservatives, so use with caution. Chlorophyll tablets can be taken during Stage 2 to lower acidity in the body and ensure a healthy acid–alkaline balance to maintain clear skin. If an adverse reaction occurs, note it in your diet diary and discontinue use.

Adult dosage: begin with one tablet daily and slowly increase the dosage according to the manufacturer's instructions. Using chlorophyll is optional.

Q & A: Chia seeds

Q: Can I eat chia seeds during the Eczema Diet?'

A: Chia seeds are tiny seeds that can be sprinkled onto breakfast cereals and porridge and they are becoming popular because of their omega-3 content. Gluten-free chia bread is also available from some health food shops. However, as they are a newly popular food with little scientific data available on them, I'm unsure of their chemical composition so I cannot add them to the eczema-safe list at present. If you want to try them, add them to your diet during Stage 2 while your skin is clear and see if you react to them. If your skin remains clear after three days, you can safely enjoy them. Linseeds/flaxseeds are an eczema-safe alternative (if you're not allergic to linseeds).

Stage 3

Stage 3 is an unofficial stage during which, if you would like to, you can add wheat and/or dairy back into your diet, and see if you can tolerate them without your eczema returning. I recommend using these products in limited amounts if you choose to do so.

Organic plain yoghurt

If you have a child recovering from eczema, they've either totally forgotten about dairy products by now or are really, really missing them. I recommend this product with some hesitancy as children can quickly become addicted to dairy products and their eczema can return. However, a small weekly, then daily serve of quality organic yoghurt can be well tolerated if your child is not allergic to dairy products. Look for these criteria when choosing yoghurt:

- must not contain natural colour 160b (annatto)
- must not contain artificial additives
- must not contain added sugar or more than 12g of sugars per 100g
- plain organic and additive-free Greek yoghurt is usually suitable
- organic vanilla yoghurt may be suitable (if no additives).

Tip: You can sweeten plain yoghurt with rice malt syrup, Banana Carob Spread, p. 220 or eczema-safe fruits.

What about cow's milk?

I have found that cow's milk (light and full cream) often causes eczema to return so you might want to delay introducing animal milks.

Wheat

When testing wheat, choose quality wheat products first such as wholemeal sourdough bread. If an adverse reaction occurs, note it in your diet diary, discontinue use and re-test the food in one to two months' time, if desired.

Chapter 18
Recipes

In your kitchen, using specially selected ingredients, you can create delicious eczema-safe meals that can improve the health of your whole body. I encourage you to make these recipes your own and experiment with the eczema-safe ingredients.

Oven temperatures

°Celsius (C)	°Fahrenheit (F)
120	250
150	300
180	355
200	400
220	450

Volume equivalents

Metric	Imperial (approximate)
20ml	½fl oz
60ml	2fl oz
80ml	3fl oz
125ml	4½fl oz
160ml	5½fl oz
180ml	6fl oz
250ml	9fl oz
375ml	13fl oz
500ml	18fl oz
750ml	1½ pints
1 litre	1¾ pint

Weight equivalents

Metric	Imperial (approximate)
10g	⅓ oz
50g	2oz
80g	3oz
100g	3½oz
150g	5oz
175g	6oz
250g	9oz
375g	13oz
500g	1lb
750g	1¾lb
1kg	2lb

Cup and spoon conversions

1 teaspoon = 5ml

1 tablespoon = 20ml

¼ cup = 60ml

⅓ cup = 80ml

½ cup = 125ml

⅔ cup = 160ml

¾ cup = 180ml

1 cup = 250ml

Symbols and abbreviations

The following is a guide to the symbols and abbreviations used throughout this book:

★	recipe or vegetable with alkalising properties
★★	recipe or vegetable with strongly alkalising properties
●	recipe or fruit rich in vitamin C and/or potassium
✱	recipe or wholegrain containing dietary fibre for gastrointestinal health
P	recipe or ingredient rich in protein and may contain iron
♦	recipe contains 1 serve of hydrating liquid
S	moderate salicylate content
SS	high to very high salicylate content
A	moderate amine content
AA	high to very high amine content
M	contains monosodium glutamate (MSG—natural or artificial flavour enhancer)
G	contains gluten
GF	gluten-free ingredient
GI	ingredient with a high glycaemic index which affects blood sugar*
Su	contains sulfites or added sulfite preservative

*If eating high GI food, take a chromium supplement once a day, or if in Stage 2 add cinnamon to the recipe to help balance blood sugar.

Breakfast

Omega Muesli ●◆❋

SERVES 1 ADULT; SOAKING TIME OVERNIGHT, PREPARATION TIME 5 MINUTES

This tasty muesli is rich in omega-3, vitamin C, potassium and fibre. Soaking the oats and linseeds overnight with ascorbic acid (pure vitamin C) or citric acid reduces the phytic acid content and increases mineral availability and goodness (using vitamin C or citric acid is optional).

½ cup rolled oats (G) (see Notes for individual measurements)
1 teaspoon whole linseeds/flaxseeds (S)
filtered water
sprinkle of ascorbic acid (or citric acid) (see 'Soaking acids', p. 80)
organic soy milk (G) or rice milk (GF) (see 'Non-dairy milks', p. 77)
½ banana, sliced (A)
1 teaspoon soy lecithin granules (if not allergic to soy)

Place oats, linseeds and water (enough to cover) into a bowl, add a sprinkle of ascorbic acid and cover with plastic wrap, then leave on the bench overnight (do not refrigerate). The next morning, drain the water using a strainer, rinse the oats and seeds with plenty of filtered water and place them in a bowl. Add rice/soy milk and top with banana and lecithin granules.

NOTES

❋ Uncooked oat measurements: for adults, use ½ cup rolled oats each; older children use ⅓ cup each, and small children ¼ cup each.

❋ You can use pear, papaya or pawpaw instead of banana.

❋ Stage 2 only: add a sprinkling of cinnamon (SS) before serving.

Surprise Porridge ●◆✳

SERVES 1 ADULT; SOAKING TIME OVERNIGHT, PREPARATION TIME 5 MINUTES, COOKING TIME 15 MINUTES

For added omega-3 goodness, add whole or freshly ground linseeds/flaxseeds to this recipe before serving (using vitamin C or citric acid is optional).

½ cup rolled oats (G) (see Notes for individual measurements)
filtered water
sprinkle of ascorbic acid or citric acid (see 'Soaking acids', p. 80)
fruit choices: peeled pear, banana (A) or papaya (A)
organic soy milk (G) or rice milk (GF) (see 'Non-dairy milks', p. 77)
1 teaspoon soy lecithin granules (if not allergic to soy)

Place oats and enough water to cover them into a bowl, add a sprinkle of ascorbic acid or citric acid (optional) and tightly cover with plastic wrap. Leave on the bench overnight. The next morning drain the water using a strainer, rinse the oats with plenty of filtered water and place them into a pot with 1½ cups filtered water (1 part oats to 3 parts water). Bring to the boil and simmer for 15 minutes, stirring occasionally. Place the fruit into an empty bowl (this is the surprise: the fruit is at the bottom). Pour on the cooked oats and top with non-dairy milk of choice, lecithin granules and extra fruit if desired.

NOTES

✸ Uncooked oat measurements: for adults, use ½ cup rolled oats each, older children use ⅓ cup each, and small children use ¼ cup each.

✸ For added omega-3, add 1 teaspoon of whole linseeds/flaxseeds before serving (soak the linseeds/flaxseeds overnight if desired).

✸ Stage 2 only: add a sprinkle of cinnamon (SS) before serving.

Quinoa Porridge GF GI 🍎 ◌ ✳

SERVES 1 ADULT; SOAKING TIME OVERNIGHT, PREPARATION TIME 5 MINUTES,
COOKING TIME 20 MINUTES

Quinoa is a nutritious gluten-free grain for those who cannot eat oat porridge.
See Notes for individual measurements (using vitamin C or citric acid is optional).

½ cup white quinoa, rinsed (do not use 'puffed' quinoa)

1 cup filtered water, plus extra for boiling

sprinkle of ascorbic acid or citric acid (see 'Soaking acids', p. 80)

½ teaspoon real vanilla essence

½ cup organic malt-free soy milk or rice milk (see 'Non-dairy milks', p. 77)

1 teaspoon whole linseeds/flaxseeds (soaked overnight if desired)

1 teaspoon rice malt syrup (optional)

fruit: papaya (A), banana (A) or peeled pear

Place the washed quinoa, water and a sprinkling of ascorbic or citric acid into a
bowl, tightly cover with plastic wrap and leave on the kitchen bench overnight.
The next morning, drain the quinoa, rinse with filtered water and place into a
saucepan. Add 1½ cups filtered water (or 3 parts water to 1 part quinoa) and
bring to the boil. Then cook over a low heat until the porridge is thick and the
grains are tender, about 20 minutes. Add the vanilla essence and milk and cook
for 5 minutes on low heat. Stir occasionally to prevent burning and add more
milk or water if necessary (you want lots of liquid to puff up the quinoa so it's very
soft). Serve with linseeds, rice malt syrup and eczema-safe fruit.

NOTES

✳ Measurements: for adults, use ½ cup quinoa each, older children use ⅓ cup
each, and small children use ¼ cup each.

✳ To reduce the phytic acid content of linseeds/flaxseeds, soak them overnight.

✳ Stage 2 only: add a sprinkle of cinnamon (SS) before serving.

Snacks

Eczema-safe Fruit Salad GF 🍎🍎

SERVES 2; PREPARATION TIME 5 MINUTES (OPTIONAL: SOAK LINSEEDS OVERNIGHT)

1 pear, peeled and diced

1 ripe banana, chopped (not sugar variety) (A)

2 slices papaya, diced (A)

1 tablespoon whole linseeds/flaxseeds (S) (soaked overnight if desired)

1 teaspoon soy lecithin granules (if not allergic to soy)

Combine all the ingredients and serve.

The Wishing Plate GF ★ ★

SERVES 2 AS A LIGHT SNACK; PREPARATION TIME 5 MINUTES

Use The Wishing Plate as a healthy and fun way to 'market' vegies to your child or simply serve these eczema-safe vegies each afternoon to help meet your alkalising vegie quota for the day. If serving to children, buy a decorative plate to use exclusively as The Wishing Plate (like it is a sacred ritual). Tell them, each time you eat a vegie from The Wishing Plate you get to make a wish. The key to inspiring children to eat vegies is to make it more convenient than other foods and to be seen eating — and visibly enjoying — vegies daily yourself. So prepare this dish each day, at around the same time to help form a habit, and leave it on the bench for everyone to snack on. Serve with Sesame-free Hummus (p. 220) if desired. Choose from the following:

1 carrot, peeled and chopped into sticks and circles (S)
1 stalk celery, strings peeled, sliced into sticks (lengthways) or 'shark's teeth'
soft green beans (blanch them for 1 minute in boiling water, allow to cool)
mung bean sprouts, thoroughly washed (remove green shells if desired)
sprouted lentils (see sprouting recipe, p. 68)

Arrange vegetables onto a fun-looking plate. Young children may want their vegies arranged into shapes (clock, truck, flower and so on), or they can create their own arrangement before eating. After eating a vegie (or sprout), make a wish.

Potato Wedges GF ★

SERVES 4; PREPARATION TIME 20 MINUTES, COOKING TIME 60 MINUTES

6–8 medium white potatoes, scrubbed (leave skin on, only peel if skin is greening)
rice bran oil, to coat
Celtic sea salt (chunky style), to taste

Preheat the oven to 200°C (400°F). Cut the potatoes into wedges. Place in a bowl and add 2 teaspoons or less of rice bran oil and mix until lightly coated. Drain off the excess oil and place the wedges on a baking tray lined with baking paper. Sprinkle with sea salt. Bake for 45–60 minutes, turning often, until wedges are browned and crispy.

NOTES

✽ Optional: sprinkle with freshly chopped parsley before serving.

✽ Stage 2 only: sprinkle on fresh rosemary, finely chopped, before baking.

Baked Banana Chips GF 🍎

SERVES 4; PREPARATION TIME 5 MINUTES, COOKING TIME 2–3 HOURS

These additive-free banana chips are naturally sweet treats that are chewy rather than crispy. You'll just need a bit of time and a pastry brush. If you have a dehydrator you can use this instead of the oven-baking method.

2 large, ripe bananas, peeled (A)
rice bran oil, to coat

Preheat the oven to 100°C (210°F) and line a baking tray with baking paper. Slice the bananas a little less than ½cm (⅛in) thick and on the diagonal (they shrink a lot so don't cut them too thin). Arrange the banana slices on the tray and brush each one on both sides with a little rice bran oil. Bake the slices for 2–3 hours, turning every half hour or so. Store them in an airtight container in the cupboard for up to 1 week.

NOTES

✽ Stage 2 only: brush on a little fresh lemon juice (SS AA) to stop them from discolouring (you may not need the rice bran oil if using lemon juice).

Dips, spreads + dressing

Bean Dip GF P ✳

SERVES 6; PREPARATION TIME 10 MINUTES (IF COOKING THE BEANS THERE IS ADDITIONAL SOAKING AND COOKING TIME)

1½ cups cooked kidney beans, see p. 86 for cooking instructions

(or use 1 x 400g/14oz can red kidney beans, drained and rinsed)

1 small clove garlic (½ teaspoon when minced)

1 tablespoon rice bran oil

⅓ teaspoon citric acid (see 'Soaking acids', p. 80)

4 tablespoons filtered water

Place all the ingredients into a blender and blend. Add extra water if necessary to make a smooth paste. Store leftovers in a sealed container in the refrigerator for up to 4 days.

Omega Salad Dressing GF SS A (Stage 2 only)

SERVES 4 ADULT-SIZED SALADS

This dressing is alkalising and makes a delicious addition to salads but it's only recommended for Stage 2 as the apple cider vinegar may cause an adverse reaction in sensitive individuals. Refer to 'Other Stage 2 additions', p. 209, for more information on apple cider vinegar.

1 tablespoon rice bran oil

2 teaspoons flaxseed oil (see Notes)

1 tablespoon apple cider vinegar (SS)(A)(Su)

2 tablespoons rice malt syrup

Place all the ingredients into a jar and shake well. Use 1 teaspoon per person on salads or baked sweet potato recipes.

NOTES

✺ Flaxseed oil changes the taste of the dressing so adjust the measurements to suit your palate. Do not use flaxseed oil on hot foods as heat damages the oil. You can also add freshly minced garlic.

Banana Carob Spread GF 🍎

MAKES 4 SERVES; PREPARATION TIME 5 MINUTES

This alkalising spread is rich in fibre and potassium. Use it on Spelt Lavash Bread (p. 229), toast, pancakes, rice crackers and so on.

1 ripe medium banana, mashed (A)

1 teaspoon carob powder

1 teaspoon rice malt syrup (optional)

sprinkle of ascorbic acid or citric acid (optional) (see 'Soaking acids', p. 80)

Mix together the banana and carob. Taste and, if desired, add rice bran syrup (for added sweetness) and ascorbic acid or citric acid (for tang) and mix. If a smooth paste is desired, blend in a small food processor. Store leftovers in a small jar and use within 2 days.

Sesame-free Hummus GF P ✳

SERVES 6; PREPARATION TIME 10 MINUTES (IF COOKING THE CHICKPEAS THERE IS ADDITIONAL SOAKING AND COOKING TIME)

This delicious hummus can be used to accompany crackers and vegie sticks; use a dollop on salads or spread it onto sandwiches or toast for a protein-rich snack, breakfast or lunch. See Notes on following page.

1½ cups cooked chickpeas (garbanzo beans)— see p. 86 for cooking instructions (or use 1 x 400g/14oz can organic chickpeas, drained and rinsed)

1 small clove garlic, minced

1 tablespoon rice bran oil

4–5 tablespoons filtered water

¼ teaspoon ascorbic acid or citric acid (see 'Soaking acids', p. 80)

¼ teaspoon Celtic sea salt

½ handful or less of chopped spring onions (scallions), green parts only

Place all the ingredients into a food processor and blend until smooth. Taste and adjust if necessary. Add a splash of water if a thinner consistency is desired. Hummus will last for 4–5 days in the refrigerator if stored in a sealed container.

NOTES

❋ This dip is wonderfully garlicky so you may want to reduce the garlic and add more after sampling.

❋ Breastfeeding: if you are breastfeeding your baby, or if your baby is windy or has colic, you may need to avoid using raw garlic and spring onions.

❋ Child: if making for a child, you may need to skip the garlic and ascorbic acid and reduce the spring onions.

Parsley Pesto GFP★
MAKES 2 SMALL JARS; PREPARATION TIME 10 MINUTES

This delicious protein-rich, alkalising spread is perfect for special occasions. Spread it onto plain rice crackers, wholegrain rye crispbread, sourdough toast and sandwiches, or add it to gluten-free pasta for a quick meal. Parsley Pesto is not suitable if you have a nut allergy of any kind and large amounts of parsley contain salicylates so eat only in moderation.

1 large bunch parsley
⅓ cup rice bran oil
1 cup unsalted raw cashews (roasted cashews are SS AA)
2 tablespoons filtered water
freshly minced garlic, to taste (begin with ½ teaspoon)
¼ teaspoon vitamin C powder or citric acid (optional, for tangy flavour)
¼ teaspoon Celtic sea salt (optional)

Cut half the stems off the parsley, wash the leaves in a bowl of water and shake off any excess water before placing them into a food processor. Add all the remaining ingredients and blend well.

NOTES

❋ Citric acid is usually found in the baking section of large supermarkets. (see 'Soaking acids', p. 80).

❋ If you would like to use less oil, use approximately 2 tablespoons rice bran oil and 3 tablespoons water.

Drinks

Healthy Skin Juice GF S★ ★ 🍎 💧

SERVES 2 ADULTS; PREPARATION TIME 5 MINUTES

This highly alkalising drink is designed to reduce inflammation, restore acid-alkaline balance in the body and aid liver detoxification of chemicals. This juice contains salicylates so if you are highly sensitive, favour Tarzan Juice below.

3 stalks celery
1–2 carrots, tops removed (S)
½ medium beetroot (S)
2 pears (must be ripe)

Wash and scrub the vegetables and peel the pears. Using a juicing machine, juice the ingredients, ending by adding a splash of filtered water.

NOTES

- Stage 2 only: add a small knob of fresh ginger, peeled (SS).

Tarzan Juice GF ★ ★ 🍎 💧

SERVES 2 ADULTS; PREPARATION TIME 5 MINUTES

This drink is low in natural chemicals and is designed to restore acid-alkaline balance in the body and aid liver detoxification of chemicals. Adjust measurements to suit your tastes.

4 stalks celery
2 large pears (must be ripe)
1–2 handfuls mung bean sprouts (freshest only, thoroughly washed)

Wash and scrub the celery and peel the pears. Using a juicing machine, juice the ingredients, ending by adding a splash of filtered water.

NOTES

- Sprouting mung beans is easy, see p. 68 for instructions. You can also use a handful of parsley in this juice.

Healthy Skin Smoothie GF 🍎◆

SERVES 2 ADULTS; PREPARATION TIME 5 MINUTES

This drink is designed to calm the itch and hydrate the skin. Pre-freeze a peeled banana to make a cold smoothie.

1 ripe banana, chopped (A) (use a frozen peeled banana)
1 slice papaya, chopped (A)
1½ cups chilled soy milk (G) or rice milk (GF) (see 'Non-dairy milks', p. 77)
1 tablespoon soy lecithin granules
1 teaspoon flaxseed oil or use ground linseeds/flaxseeds
splash of real vanilla essence

Place all the ingredients into a blender and blend on high until smooth.

NOTES
✹ You can add 1 sprig of parsley, finely chopped, for alkalising.
✹ Stage 2 only: add a sprinkling of cinnamon for blood sugar balance.

Flaxseed Lemon Drink GF SS AA Stage 2 only ★ ★ ◆

SERVES 2 ADULTS; PREPARATION TIME 5 MINUTES

Over the years I've had such great feedback about this Healthy Skin Diet alkalising drink (this is a simplified version). The pectin and oils from lemon skin provide antioxidants, chelate toxins from the bowel and stimulate liver detoxification enzymes. The lecithin aids fat digestion and helps the body utilise the anti-inflammatory omega-3 oils. A word of caution: this drink is only suitable for those who are not sensitive to salicylates or amines, as lemon is rich in both.

½ lemon, skin washed and scrubbed (SS)(AA)
2 cups chilled filtered water
1 tablespoon soy lecithin granules
2 teaspoons organic flaxseed oil (S)

Finely grate (zest) the skin of the lemon and place into a blender. Then add the juice of the lemon and the remaining ingredients. Blend on high for 30 seconds or until frothy and thoroughly blended. Strain if desired. Have this drink throughout the day or before each main meal.

Baby food

Teething Rusks GF 🍎 ☀

MAKES 20+; COOKING TIME 1–2 HOURS

1 cup mashed banana (A)
1 cup rice flour (brown if available)
filtered water

Preheat the oven to 150°C (300°F). Using a food processor, purée the banana then add the flour and mix together on low speed. Add water if necessary, 1 teaspoon at a time, to make a stiff, dryish dough (do not make it wet).

On a floured board, roll out the mixture into long, thin sausages, then slice into 8cm (3in) lengths. Line a baking tray with baking paper and bake the rusks for 1–1½ hours or until they are hard (this may take up to 2 hours, depending on how much liquid you have used). Store in an airtight container for up to 1 week.

NOTES

❀ You can substitute the banana with 1 cup stewed pear, mashed, or any other eczema-safe fruit or vegetable such as 1 cup cooked sweet potato (S), swede (rutabaga) or carrot (S).

❀ Ensure that the rusks bake hard.

❀ When feeding your infant teething rusks, finger foods or any other food that could be a choking hazard, it's important to supervise your child and ensure they are sitting upright.

Bean Face on Rice GF ★ ☀ P

SERVES 2 SMALL CHILDREN; PREPARATION TIME 10 MINUTES

½ cup cooked rice, warm
½ cup cooked chickpeas (garbanzo beans) (cooking instructions, p. 86)
2 cooked green beans or 2 pieces of celery, chopped
4 carrot slices (S)

Place the warm rice in a bowl and arrange the chickpeas and vegetables to make a smiling face or a clock face.

Lunch + dinner

Alkaline Vegie Broth GF ★ ◆

MAKES 6–8 CUPS OF BROTH; PREPARATION TIME 15 MINUTES,
COOKING TIME 1½ HOURS

A nutritious, alkaline vegetarian and vegan broth, rich in flavonoids and antioxidants. Use it to flavour soups and casseroles.

½ leek, finely sliced

4 cloves garlic, minced

3 stalks celery, chopped

3 brussels sprouts, chopped

3 potatoes (with skins if not going green), scrubbed and diced

1 handful parsley

2½ litres (5 pints) filtered water

1 teaspoon Celtic sea salt

pinch of ascorbic acid (optional) (see 'Soaking acids', p. 80)

In a stockpot or very large saucepan, heat a splash of water on medium heat and sauté the leek and garlic for 5 minutes. Add the remaining ingredients to the pot, cover and bring to the boil. Reduce the heat to low and simmer for 1–2 hours, stirring occasionally. Remove from the heat and allow to cool for a few minutes. Strain the broth, using a spatula or measuring cup to press out the liquid from the vegetables. Discard the strained vegetables.

NOTES

❋ Broth will last for a week if refrigerated. Store the leftover broth in clean glass jars or containers, and freeze the leftovers: most soup/casserole recipes use 3 cups of broth so measure portions of 3 cups each and write the volume on the container before freezing, and freeze 1 tablespoon portions in ice-cube trays for use in pasta dishes or children's meals.

❋ Stage 2 only: ½ teaspoon grated fresh ginger root (SS) and 1 bay leaf (S).

Therapeutic Broth GF ★ ★ ◆ AA

MAKES 6–8 CUPS OF BROTH; PREPARATION TIME 10 MINUTES,
COOKING TIME 6.5 HOURS, MAKE 1 DAY BEFORE USE.

This alkaline broth is rich in glycine, collagen, calcium and magnesium. It boosts liver detoxification and can reduce inflammation and strengthen the immune system if you have a cold or flu (thanks to the cysteine). The secret to a therapeutic broth is the addition of a weak acid, such as citric acid or ascorbic acid (pure vitamin C powder), to draw out the minerals from the bones.

Use this broth as a drink when you are ill, or as a tasty stock in casseroles and soups. If you have amine sensitivity use Alkaline Vegie Broth instead.

2 large beef bones, with a little meat on them (including necks, joints, marrow, lamb bones)
3½ litres (7½ pints) filtered water (room temperature, not heated)
1 large or 2 small free-range/organic chicken carcasses
¼ teaspoon ascorbic acid or citric acid (see 'Soaking acids', p. 80)
½ large leek (white parts)
2 spring onions (scallions), ends trimmed
2 brussels sprouts
2 stalks celery
1 white potato (use skins if not going green)
3–4 cloves garlic, minced
1 teaspoon Celtic sea salt

Preheat the oven to 200°C (400°F). In a roasting pan, roast the beef bones for 30 minutes or until deliciously fragrant and browned. Remove from the oven and add them to a stockpot or very large saucepan along with the water, chicken carcasses and ascorbic acid or citric acid. Cover, bring to the boil and then simmer on low heat (do not add the vegetables yet). Meanwhile, wash, scrub and chop the vegies into small pieces.

After 1–2 hours of cooking, break apart the carcasses using tongs, to allow more of the minerals to be extracted from the bones. Add the chopped vegetables and the remaining ingredients. Cook for a total of 6 hours. The broth is more flavoursome if it reduces almost by half.

Remove the bones (the chicken bones should be soft and should crumble when squeezed). Place a strainer over a large bowl then pour the broth through the strainer, discarding the boiled bones and vegetables when you have finished. Squeeze out as much liquid as possible as you strain the broth (press a measuring cup on the cooked meat and vegetables to squeeze out the remaining liquid).

The next step is very important: store the broth in a sealed container in the refrigerator overnight so the fat has time to solidify. The next day carefully lift or skim off the layer of fat (this saturated fat is no good for your eczema). If your broth is thick and jelly-like, it means it's rich in collagen (gelatin).

NOTES

- Broth will last for a week if refrigerated and used in soups etc. Store the leftover broth in clean glass jars or containers, and freeze the leftovers: most soup/casserole recipes use 3 cups of broth so measure out portions of 3 cups each and write the volume on the container before freezing, and freeze 1 tablespoon portions into icecube trays (cover with plastic wrap) for use in pasta dishes and children's meals.

Design Your Own Sandwich *

Eczema-safe sandwiches and wraps are great for lunches and snacks. Here are your options.

Bread choices

spelt sourdough (G) (available from some health food shops)
   Spelt Lavash Bread, p. 229
gluten-free bread (check the ingredients are eczema-safe)
multigrain/wholegrain rye crispbread (check there are no trans fats)

Spread choices

Sesame-free Hummus, p. 220
Parsley Pesto, p. 221 (in moderation, not daily)
Bean Dip, p. 219
Banana Carob Spread, p. 220
pure organic butter (Stage 2 only and allergy permitting)

Sandwich fillings

skinless cooked chicken and mung bean sprouts (P)★
trout, salmon or tuna (A)(P), grated carrot (S) and iceberg lettuce s
home-cooked or organic turkey breast* and cos (romaine) lettuce (S)(P)★
sliced lean roast lamb and leftover roast vegetables (P)★
iceberg lettuce, mung bean sprouts, grated carrot (S) and grated beetroot (S)★ ★
banana (A) and rice malt syrup (occasionally) ★ ★
mashed boiled egg and iceberg lettuce (P)★ (allergy permitting and preferably in
   Stage 2)

NOTES

❀ *Only use organic or home-cooked meats as pre-sliced or deli meats contain
   flavour enhancers and may contain irritating preservatives such as nitrates.

Quinoa 'Rice' GF GI ✸

SERVES 1 ADULT; SOAKING TIME OVERNIGHT, PREPARATION TIME 5 MINUTES, COOKING TIME 15–20 MINUTES

Quinoa is a nutritious gluten-free grain for those who cannot eat oats, wheat and other gluten-rich grains. Use as a rice substitute or make into porridge.

½ cup white quinoa, rinsed (do not use 'puffed' quinoa)
1 cup filtered water for soaking (room temperature), plus 1½ cups extra for cooking
sprinkle of ascorbic acid or citric acid (optional, see 'Soaking acids', p. 80)

Place the washed quinoa, water and ascorbic acid or citric acid into a bowl, cover with plastic wrap and leave on the kitchen bench overnight. The next morning, drain the quinoa, rinse it and place it into a small saucepan, add the extra of filtered water and bring to the boil. Cook over low heat until the mixture is thick and the grains are tender, about 20 minutes.

Spelt Lavash Bread (or Spelt Chips) ✸

MAKES 6 FLAT WRAPS; PREPARATION TIME 8 MINUTES, RESTING TIME 30 MINUTES, COOKING TIME 20 MINUTES

This flat bread is delicious and easy to make. For topping suggestions, refer to Design Your Own Sandwich, p. 228. For instructions on how to make Spelt Chips read the notes at the end of this recipe.

1¼ cups plain spelt flour, plus extra (wholemeal if available) (G)
¾ teaspoon finely ground Celtic sea salt
1 tablespoon rice bran oil
⅔ cup boiling hot water

In a bowl, mix the spelt flour and the salt. Add the rice bran oil and the hot water and mix using a knife. Lightly flour your chopping board and knead the dough for approximately 3 minutes until smooth and elastic. Cut into 6 balls. Place onto a plate, cover with plastic wrap and rest for 30 minutes.

On a floured board, roll each ball with a rolling pin to make large thin circles. Heat a large non-stick frying pan over high heat and cook each flat bread for 1 minute each side, or until bubbles appear and the bread becomes browned in spots. Turn down the heat if necessary to avoid burning. For soft wraps, cook them quickly. (Thanks Bianca Rothwell for supplying this recipe.)

NOTES

❀ How to make spelt chips: roll each ball of dough until it is very thin. Then cut out triangles and bake in the oven (preheated to 180°C/355°F) until crisp.

Papaya Rice Paper Rolls GF P ★ ●

SERVES 4 (MAKES 20 ROLLS); PREPARATION TIME 40 MINUTES

This recipe gets ★ ★ if using mung bean sprouts.

500g (1lb) skinless free-range chicken, thinly sliced
freshly minced garlic or dried garlic powder, to taste
Celtic sea salt (optional), to taste
packet of round rice paper (20 sheets or 250g/9oz)
½ ripe papaya (A), skin and seeds discarded, thinly sliced
3 handfuls cos (romaine) or iceberg lettuce, finely shredded
2 medium carrots, grated (S)
mung bean sprouts (freshest only), washed

Season the chicken with a sprinkling of garlic and salt and place in a steamer. Steam the chicken for 5 minutes or until thoroughly cooked. Remove from the heat and allow to partially cool. Wet a clean tea towel, wring out the excess water and place flat on a bench. Soften the rice paper, one sheet at a time, in a large bowl of very warm water, soaking each one for 10–20 seconds. Remove the rice paper before it gets too soft and place flat on the damp tea towel. Arrange a variety of ingredients (in a row) on the rice paper near the end closest to you, then roll it up, tucking the ends in about halfway so they look like cylinders (also refer to the rice paper packaging for instructions).

NOTES

❀ Stage 2 only: add chopped fresh mint.

Chickpea Rice GFP ★ ✹

SERVES 2 (OR 4 WHEN SERVING WITH MEAT OR FISH);
PREPARATION TIME 15 MINUTES, COOKING TIME 30 MINUTES

1 small to medium sweet potato, scrubbed (S)

rice bran oil, to coat

1½ cups basmati rice (or 2½ cups brown rice; see Notes)

4–5 spring onions (scallions), chopped (children might prefer these well cooked/ fried)

3 tablespoons Therapeutic Broth (p. 226; V&Vn: use Alkaline Vegie Broth, p. 225)

1½ cups cooked chickpeas (garbanzo beans)(see p. 86 for cooking instructions) or use 1 x 400g (14oz) can organic chickpeas, drained and rinsed

1 handful mung bean sprouts, thoroughly washed

1 handful flat-leaf (Italian) parsley, washed and chopped

1 handful raw cashews (optional and allergy permitting)

If the skin of the sweet potato is undamaged keep it on, or peel if necessary. Cut the sweet potatoes in half lengthways and then into wedges. Either steam the sweet potato for 10 minutes (this is the healthiest option) or roast in the oven: preheat the oven to 200°C (400°F), then in a bowl, coat the wedges in a little rice bran oil, sprinkle with Celtic sea salt (optional) and drain most of the oil off before roasting the pieces on a tray lined with baking paper. This will take about 30 minutes or until soft. Meanwhile, boil the rice for 10 minutes or according to the packet instructions (brown rice takes approx. 25 minutes). Drain.

In a frying pan, lightly sauté the spring onions in the broth, add the chickpeas and cooked rice and briefly heat. Place in shallow bowls and top with the sweet potato, mung bean sprouts, parsley and raw cashews.

NOTES

✹ Do not use 'quick' or 'instant' brown rice. Brown rice has a high GI so use basmati or doongara rice if you have blood sugar problems such as diabetes.

Roasted Potato Stack GF P ★ ★ ✹

SERVES 2; PREPARATION TIME 10 MINUTES, COOKING TIME 30 MINUTES

This nutritious snack is rich in alkalising vegetables and balanced with protein (if using fish and/or hummus). If you are vegetarian or vegan omit the fish.

4 large white potatoes (or 2 small sweet potatoes)
½ teaspoon rice bran oil
1 piece flathead or other eczema-safe fish or 1 x 95g (3½oz) can tuna, quality chunky style in springwater or brine
dried garlic powder, to taste
Celtic sea salt, to taste
2 dollops Sesame-free Hummus, p. 220
1 handful mung bean sprouts, thoroughly washed (freshest only; see 'Sprouting recipe', p. 68)

Preheat the oven to 200°C (400°F). Scrub the potatoes in water and keep the skins on if they're not greening (peel any green bits). Cut them in half lengthways, coat them in a little rice bran oil and roast on a baking tray lined with baking paper for 30–40 minutes or until very soft.

Halve the fish, rub a drop or two of rice bran oil onto the fish and sprinkle it with dried garlic powder and Celtic sea salt if desired. Bake the fish alongside the potatoes for the last 10–12 minutes.

Remove the potatoes and fish from the oven. Put the hummus on top of the potatoes and sprinkle with mung bean sprouts and serve beside the fish.

Roasted Sweet Potato Salad GF P ★ ★ ✽

SERVES 2; PREPARATION TIME 10 MINUTES, COOKING TIME 30 MINUTES

½ teaspoon rice bran oil
1 small to medium sweet potato, peeled and diced (S)
Celtic sea salt, to taste
1 quantity Sesame-free Hummus, p. 220
cos (romaine) lettuce leaves (or iceberg lettuce), torn
1 handful mung bean sprouts, thoroughly washed
sprinkling of unsalted raw cashews (optional)

Preheat the oven to 200°C (400°F). Lightly oil the potato with a little rice bran oil (do not let the potato sit in oil) and sprinkle with salt. Roast the potato for 30 minutes or until very soft on the inside. Meanwhile, make the Sesame-free Hummus if not already made. Arrange the salad leaves onto a plate. Add the sweet potato and serve with a dollop of hummus and top with sprouts and cashews.

NOTES

✽ Stage 2 only: add a teaspoon of delicious Omega Salad Dressing (p. 219) if you are not sensitive to sulfites (refer to apple cider vinegar information, p. 209).

Alkaline Bomb Salad GF ★ ★

SERVES 2; PREPARATION TIME 10 MINUTES

4 handfuls (approx. 200g/7oz) iceberg or cos (romaine) lettuce, torn
1 small stalk celery, chopped
1–2 spring onions (scallions), thinly sliced on the diagonal
1–2 handfuls mung bean sprouts, freshest only, washed
Sesame-free Hummus (p. 220) or Bean Dip (p. 219)

Place the lettuce into two shallow serving bowls and top with the remaining ingredients, finishing with a large dollop of hummus or dip.

New Potato and Leek Soup GF P ★ ★ ◆

MAKES 6-8 SERVES; PREPARATION TIME 20 MINUTES, COOKING TIME 30 MINUTES

2 large leeks, green parts removed, finely sliced

2 cloves garlic, minced

3 cups Therapeutic Broth, p. 226 (V&Vn: use Alkaline Vegie Broth, p. 225

6 cups filtered water

1.2kg (2½lb) white potatoes (8 medium to large potatoes, preferably carisma/low
    GI, see Resources, p. 265)

4 brussels sprouts, diced

¼ cup fresh parsley

½ teaspoon Celtic sea salt (optional)

In a stockpot or very large saucepan, heat a splash of water on medium heat and lightly fry the leeks and garlic. Add the broth and water, cover and bring to the boil.

Meanwhile, peel and chop the potatoes and add them to the pot along with the brussels sprouts. Cover and bring to the boil. Reduce the heat to low and simmer for 20–30 minutes, stirring occasionally. Remove from the heat, uncover and allow to cool for 5 minutes.

Chop the parsley leaves and discard the stems. Add the parsley and Celtic sea salt to the soup.

One batch at a time, process the soup in a blender or food processor until smooth. The soup should have a thick consistency. If the soup is too thick, add more water.

NOTES

❋ Add extra water the next day if the soup thickens overnight.

Sunshine Soup GF S ★ ★ ◆

MAKES 6–7 SERVES; PREPARATION TIME 20 MINUTES, COOKING TIME 30 MINUTES

3 cups Therapeutic Broth, p. 226 (V&Vn: use Alkaline Vegie Broth, p. 225)

4–5 cups filtered water

1.2 kg (2½lb) sweet potatoes (see Notes) (S)

2 cloves garlic, minced

3 brussels sprouts, finely chopped

1 leek, green part removed, finely chopped

Celtic sea salt, to taste

1 handful chopped parsley (optional), to serve

Place the Therapeutic Broth and water in a stockpot or large saucepan, cover with a lid and bring to the boil. Peel and chop the sweet potatoes and add them to the soup along with the garlic, brussels sprouts and leek. Cover and simmer for 25 minutes. Taste and add salt if desired.

Remove the saucepan from the heat, uncover and allow the soup to cool for 5 minutes. Using a blender or food processor, blend the soup in batches to make a smooth soup. Add another ½ cup or more of water if necessary. Serve in bowls and top with chopped parsley.

NOTES

❀ 1.2kg (2½lb) of sweet potato is approximately 4 large sweet potatoes (S), or if you want fewer salicylates use 2 sweet potatoes and 5 medium white potatoes (peeled).

Country Chicken Soup S P ★ ❋ ◈

MAKES 8 SERVES; PREPARATION TIME 10 MINUTES (SOAKING BARLEY OVERNIGHT RECOMMENDED), COOKING TIME 25 MINUTES OR 45 MINUTES IF THE BARLEY HAS NOT BEEN SOAKED

3 cups Therapeutic Broth, p. 226 (**V&Vn: use Alkaline Vegie Broth, p. 225**)

2 litres (4 pints) filtered water

2 cloves garlic, minced

400g (14 oz) skinless chicken or 4 chicken thigh fillets, finely diced

1 large carrot, finely diced (S)

2 stalks celery, cut lengthways and finely diced

2 spring onions (scallions), finely chopped

2 brussels sprouts, finely diced

¼–½ teaspoon Celtic sea salt, optional

½ cup barley (G), rinsed, preferably soaked overnight (see 'How to soak grains' p. 80)

Place the broth and water into a stockpot or large saucepan, bring to the boil and add the remaining ingredients. Cover and simmer for 25 minutes (or 45 minutes if the barley has not been soaked).

NOTES

❋ Variations include adding finely chopped leeks or cabbage and chopped parsley to garnish when serving. Add extra vegetables if a heartier soup is desired.

❋ Stage 2 only: add a sprinkling of grated fresh ginger (SS) and you can use a heaped teaspoon of organic vegetable stock powder if desired.

Baked Fish with Mash **s p ★ ★**

SERVES 2 ADULTS AND 2 CHILDREN; PREPARATION TIME 10 MINUTES, COOKING TIME 25 MINUTES

1 sweet potato, peeled and diced (S)

3 white potatoes, peeled and diced

splash organic soy milk (G) (see 'Non-dairy milks', p. 77)

Celtic sea salt (optional), to taste

trout fillets (½ fillet each adult, see Notes), halved lengthways

rice bran oil, to coat

1 small handful flat-leaf (Italian) parsley, washed and chopped, stems removed

dried garlic powder, to taste

3 handfuls green beans, ends trimmed

4 brussels sprouts

Preheat the oven to 200°C (400°F). Steam the sweet potato and potato over a steamer using a little water, for 15 minutes or until very soft (reserve the water for steaming the greens). Mash the potato, stir through the soy milk (you may need ¼ cup), sprinkle with Celtic sea salt if desired and set aside.

Place the fish in a baking dish lined with baking paper, lightly coat it with rice bran oil and top with parsley and dried garlic powder. Bake for 10 minutes or until cooked to your liking (times will vary depending on the thickness of the fish so check it after 8 minutes). Steam the greens until tender and reheat the mash before serving.

NOTES

✸ If you are vegetarian or vegan use lentils, tofu, chickpeas (garbanzo beans) or beans instead of fish. For a creamy mash add soy milk. For a gluten-free meal use malt-free soy milk, rice milk or Therapeutic Broth (p. 226) in the mash (V&Vn: use Alkaline Vegie Broth, p. 225).

✸ Each serving size of fish should be around the size of the palm of your hand. Fish is usually sold in large pieces so you will probably only need half of one fillet per adult.

✸ If the fish develops white clumps on the sides during cooking it's overcooking so remove immediately from the oven.

Sticks and Stones (fish or chicken on skewers)
GF P ★

SERVES 2 ADULTS AND 2 CHILDREN; PREPARATION TIME 30 MINUTES,
COOKING TIME 10 MINUTES

12–14 bamboo skewers

approx. 600g (1⅓lb) boneless trout fillets (AA) or skinless chicken thigh fillets
(preferably free range or organic)

3 large spring onions (scallions), chopped into 2cm (¾in) pieces

dried garlic powder, to taste

Celtic sea salt (optional), to taste

Alkaline Bomb Salad, p. 233, to serve

Preheat the oven to 200°C (400°F). Soak the bamboo skewers in water for at least 15 minutes to prevent them from burning during cooking. Line a baking tray with baking paper. Cut the trout or chicken into 2cm (¾in) cubes and in alternating patterns, thread it and the spring onions onto the skewers, leaving a 5cm (2in) space at the blunt end of each skewer. Place on the baking tray and season with dried garlic powder and Celtic sea salt. Bake the skewers in the oven for 10 minutes or until thoroughly cooked.

Meanwhile, prepare the Alkaline Bomb Salad and serve it alongside the warm skewers.

NOTES

❋ If you would like a heavier meal, serve with basmati rice or brown rice (GI). Do not use 'quick' or 'instant' brown rice. Brown rice has a high GI so use basmati or doongara rice if you have blood sugar problems such as diabetes.

❋ V&Vn: If you are vegetarian or vegan, use firm tofu.

Eczema-safe Gravy GF

SERVES 6+; PREPARATION TIME 5 MINUTES (BROTH NEEDS TO BE PRE-MADE),
COOKING TIME 10–15 MINUTES

This basic gravy is a perfect accompaniment for roasts and meat dishes. If you are allergic to rice, use spelt flour or another eczema-safe flour, listed on p. 82.

1 cup Therapeutic Broth, p. 226
2 teaspoons rice flour (brown if available)
sprinkling of dried garlic powder
pinch of Celtic sea salt

Place the broth into a small saucepan on high heat, bring to the boil then reduce to a simmer. In a cup, mix the rice flour with 1–2 tablespoons of cool filtered water and when it's lump-free add it to the broth and mix until it begins to thicken. Taste and add dried garlic powder and a pinch of salt if desired.

Smashed Potato s ★

SERVES 4; PREPARATION TIME 10 MINUTES, COOKING TIME 15 MINUTES

4–6 large white potatoes, peeled and diced
1 small to medium sweet potato, peeled and diced (S)
¼ cup organic soy milk (G) or rice milk (GF)
Celtic sea salt, to taste

In a saucepan, boil or steam the potatoes and sweet potato until soft (approximately 15 minutes). Drain and return the potatoes to the saucepan, then add the milk and salt and mash.

Easy Roast Chicken GF S P ★

SERVES 4 WITH LEFTOVERS FOR A SECOND MEAL; PREPARATION TIME 10 MINUTES, COOKING TIME 1½ HOURS (ALLOW 15 MINUTES TO PREHEAT THE OVEN)

You can steam the vegies instead of roasting and serve this meal with Eczema-safe Gravy (p. 239). If possible, use a deep baking dish that has a wire rack at the bottom.

1 x 1.8kg (4lb) whole chicken
rice bran oil, to coat
sprinkling of Celtic sea salt
dried garlic powder, to taste
8 potatoes (or enough for family)
4 carrots, sliced on diagonal (S)
½ sweet potato, peeled and sliced (S)
4 brussels sprouts
2 handfuls green beans, ends trimmed

Preheat the oven to 200°C (400°F). Rinse the chicken both inside and out and pat the outside dry with a paper towel. Rub rice bran oil over the chicken and then sprinkle with salt and dried garlic powder. Place the chicken upside down in a large, deep ovenproof dish with a wire rack inside so the chicken and the spare vegies don't sit in the oil. For an extra tender roast and if using a wire rack, place 1 cup of water into the bottom of the dish (ensuring the water does not touch the chicken). Cook the chicken for 30 minutes before turning it right side up.

Meanwhile, peel the potatoes if the skin is greening. Chop the potatoes into chunks and place them, along with the sliced carrots and sweet potato, into a large bowl and drizzle with a little rice bran oil, ensuring to drain off the excess oil. Place the potato, carrot and sweet potato on a large tray lined with baking paper and sprinkle with Celtic sea salt (if more space is needed, some of these can cook beside the chicken on the wire rack). Place the vegetable tray into the oven. Roast for 1 hour, turning the vegies regularly. Roast until the chicken is thoroughly cooked and no longer pink inside (check around the drumsticks by gently pulling the flesh away from the bone). Cook for a further 10 minutes if necessary.

In the last 10 minutes, make the gravy, if desired, and heat up 2½cm (1in) of water in the base of a saucepan/steamer and steam the brussels sprouts for 6 minutes and the beans for 3–4 minutes.

NOTES

- Use leftover chicken meat to make Country Chicken Soup, p. 236.

Cinnamon Chicken **GF SS P ★ ★**

SERVES 2 ADULTS AND 2 CHILDREN; PREPARATION TIME 25 MINUTES, COOKING TIME 15 MINUTES

If using this recipe during Stage 1, omit the cinnamon and use Celtic sea salt and dried parsley flakes instead.

1 teaspoon rice bran oil
2 cloves garlic, minced
¼ teaspoon ground cinnamon (SS)
500g (1lb) free-range chicken breast or thigh, finely sliced, fat removed
5 medium spring onions (scallions), chopped
4 large white potatoes, scrubbed and chopped (peel skin if greening)
1 small to medium sweet potato (S), peeled and chopped
6 brussels sprouts, finely sliced (or use green beans)
2 handfuls mung bean sprouts, thoroughly washed
Celtic sea salt (optional)

In a bowl, mix the rice bran oil with the garlic and cinnamon then add the chicken pieces and mix. Stir-fry the chicken in a non-stick pan on medium–high heat and add the spring onions for the last 1–2 minutes of cooking. Ensure the chicken is thoroughly cooked.

Meanwhile, steam the potato, sweet potato and brussels sprouts until soft. Serve topped with mung bean sprouts and a sprinkling of Celtic sea salt if desired.

Chickpea Casserole GF P ★ ★ ✹

SERVES 6; PREPARATION TIME 20 MINUTES, COOKING TIME 1 HOUR

3 cups Therapeutic Broth, p. 226 (V&Vn: use Alkaline Vegie Broth, p. 225)

1 cup filtered water (or use 1 extra cup Therapeutic Broth)

1–2 teaspoons brown rice flour (GF) or spelt flour (contains gluten)

2½ cups cooked chickpeas (garbanzo beans) (cooking instructions, p. 86) or use
    2 x 400g (14oz) cans organic chickpeas, drained and rinsed

4 medium potatoes, scrubbed and diced (peel skin if greening)

1 medium to large sweet potato, peeled and diced (S)

1 leek, finely chopped

4 brussels sprouts, finely sliced

4 stalks celery, halved lengthways and finely chopped

2 cloves garlic, minced

chopped parsley, to garnish (optional)

spring onions (scallions), to garnish (optional)

Preheat the oven to 200°C (400°F). Place the broth and water into a large casserole dish. In a cup, mix the flour with a little water until there are no lumps then add it to the broth and mix. Rinse the chickpeas and discard any discoloured ones, then add them to the broth. Add the remaining ingredients and cook for 1 hour, stirring occasionally. The casserole should be slightly soupy so add extra water if necessary. Garnish with chopped parsley or spring onions if desired.

NOTES

✹ Variations: add chopped spring onions (scallions), swedes (rutabaga) and skinless chicken instead of chickpeas (during the 3-day Alkalising Cleanse don't use chicken and preferably don't use flour).

✹ Stage 2 only: you can add a little organic stock powder to see if you can tolerate it (it may contain salicylates and natural MSG). If you can tolerate it well and you don't have eczema, you can use a quality, all natural stock powder and water instead of the broth if you are short on time. Or you can add a sprinkling of cinnamon and/or cumin if you have tested them and tolerate them well.

My Favourite Lamb Cutlets GF P ★

SERVES 4 (2 ADULTS AND 2 CHILDREN); PREPARATION TIME 10 MINUTES, COOKING TIME 40 MINUTES

2 tablespoons Parsley Pesto, p. 221 (if not allergic to nuts)

rice bran oil

8 Frenched lamb cutlets (with fat trimmed or use lean lamb fillets)

Celtic sea salt (optional), to taste

4–6 large potatoes, scrubbed and chopped (peel if skin is greening)

8 brussels sprouts, ends trimmed

2 handfuls green beans, ends trimmed

Preheat the oven to 240°C (460°F). (You can grill the cutlets if preferred.) If you haven't already made the Parsley Pesto, make it now.

Heat a splash of oil in a frying pan on high heat, coat the lamb cutlets in a little oil and sprinkle with Celtic sea salt if desired. When the pan is hot, seal the cutlets for 1 minute on each side. Remove from the heat. Line a shallow baking dish or tray with baking paper, then place the cutlets in the dish and roast for 5 minutes. Turn once and spread a thick layer of pesto on the top side of the cutlets and return to the oven to cook for a further 5 minutes or until cooked to your liking.

Meanwhile, bring a saucepan of water to the boil and steam the potatoes for 10–15 minutes. In the last 3–5 minutes of cooking, add the brussels sprouts and beans to the steamer and cook until soft.

Pasta GF P ✳ ★

SERVES 2 ADULTS; PREPARATION TIME 15 MINUTES (25 MINUTES IF MAKING PESTO), COOKING TIME 15 MINUTES

This is a basic pasta recipe that you can modify if desired.

350g (12oz) skinless chicken, lean lamb or eczema-safe fish, p. 72 (V&Vn: use kidney beans)

2 teaspoons rice bran oil

2 cloves garlic, minced

½ bunch spring onions (scallions), chopped

3 handfuls green beans, ends trimmed and sliced

250g (8⅔oz) gluten-free pasta or buckwheat pasta (GF)

4–5 tablespoons Therapeutic Broth, p. 226 (V&Vn: Alkaline Vegie Broth, p. 225)

Celtic sea salt, to taste

Parsley Pesto, p. 221 (if no allergy to nuts)

Dice or slice the chicken, lamb or fish and drizzle with 1 teaspoon of rice bran oil, then sprinkle with the garlic and mix to coat. In a large non-stick frying pan, stir-fry the fish or meat until cooked to your liking. Remove from the heat and cover to keep it warm. Clean the pan then add the remaining rice bran oil, and the spring onions and green beans, and lightly fry.

Meanwhile, cook the pasta according to the packet instructions. Drain and add the pasta to the frying pan and mix it with the spring onions and beans. Add enough broth to stop the pasta from going dry, and season with a little Celtic sea salt. Divide the pasta into 2 serving bowls and top with the meat or fish, then add a dollop of Parsley Pesto on top of each serving.

Sweet treats

Choco Milk (hot or cold)◆

SERVES 1 ADULT OR 2 CHILDREN

This tasty carob drink is caffeine-free and suitable as an occasional treat.

½ teaspoon carob powder
1½ cups organic soy milk or rice milk (GF) (see 'Non-dairy milks', p. 77)
1 teaspoon rice malt syrup (optional, it may not need sweetening)

Cold chocolate milk: The secret to a lump-free drink is to mix the carob powder in a teaspoon of boiling hot water before adding it to the milk. Taste and sweeten it with rice malt syrup if desired. Alternatively, combine all the ingredients in a blender and blend on high until smooth.

Hot chocolate: Heat the milk in a small saucepan over medium heat. Once the milk is warm (or hot, if desired), add the remaining ingredients and stir.

Banana Icy Poles GF 🍎

SERVES 4; PREPARATION TIME 5 MINUTES, ALLOW FOR FREEZING TIME

1 large ripe banana, mashed (A)
½ cup+ rice milk

Mix the two ingredients together, using a splash of rice milk at a time, until you achieve the desired consistency. Freeze in a plastic iceblock (popsicle/ice lolly) mould and serve once hard (it's best to let them set overnight).

NOTES

❋ You can also add rice malt syrup, real vanilla essence or a sprinkle of carob powder.

Birthday Cake GF

SERVES 10; PREPARATION TIME 10 MINUTES, COOKING TIME 30 MINUTES

This dairy-free, gluten-free vanilla cake is for people who are sensitive to dairy and gluten. Preferably use a cake tin that has a hole in the middle. Give your cake the wow factor by using a 24cm (9½in) fluted cake tin — the kind that makes a hole in the centre and jelly-mould ridges around the sides. These are available from large department stores and speciality kitchen shops. You can use this cake recipe to make gluten-free cupcakes (medium-sized cupcakes cook in 10 minutes). See Notes for variations and icing.

2¼ cups gluten-free self-raising flour
    (e.g. White Wings Gluten Free Self Raising Flour)
¾ cup fine raw sugar
½ teaspoon bicarbonate of soda (baking soda)
¾ cup organic rice milk (see 'Non-dairy milks', p. 77)
2 free-range eggs or equivalent egg replacer
½ teaspoon real vanilla essence
¼ cup rice bran oil

Preheat the oven to 180°C (355°F). Using rice bran oil, oil a fluted cake tin or a round cake tin. In a mixing bowl combine the flour, sugar and bicarbonate of soda. In a food processor, blend the rice milk, eggs and vanilla essence. Then, while the motor is running, open the shute and slowly drizzle in the oil and blend well until smooth and creamy. Add the dry ingredients to the wet and mix on low speed (or with a wooden spoon) until smooth. Pour the mixture into the prepared cake tin and bake for 20–30 minutes or until cooked (if the tin has a hole in the centre cooking time will be closer to 20 minutes). Test with a wooden skewer to see if the middle is cooked through; the skewer should come out clean.

Allow to cool for 5 minutes before removing the cake from the tin. Store at room temperature for up to 24 hours (cakes are softer if not refrigerated before the party), and store leftovers in a sealed container in the refrigerator.

NOTES

❀ To ice this cake, use gluten-free icing sugar mixed with a little water (drizzle or spread it on), or dust the top of the cake with gluten-free icing sugar.

Spelt Pancakes ✳ 🍅P

SERVES 2 ADULTS — MAKES 6–8 PANCAKES; PREPARATION TIME 5 MINUTES,
COOKING TIME 15 MINUTES

Spelt pancakes taste very similar to wheat pancakes and they make a great dessert or snack. The gluten-free version is Buckwheat Crepes (see p. 248).

1 cup spelt flour (G) (wholemeal if available)

¼ teaspoon bicarbonate of soda (baking soda)

1¼ cups organic soy milk (G) (see 'Non-dairy milks', p. 77)

1 egg, lightly beaten (or egg-free equivalent)

rice bran oil, to coat the pan

rice malt syrup, to serve

1–2 bananas, sliced (A) (or papaya), to serve

In a mixing bowl, combine the flour and bicarbonate of soda and sift if necessary. Gradually mix in the milk and stir until lump-free, then stir in the egg. Heat a small non-stick frying pan, add a little oil and using a ⅓ measuring cup, pour the mixture into the pan. Lightly cook each side. Repeat until all the mixture has been used.

Spread a thin layer of rice malt syrup onto the pancakes and top with eczema-safe fruit.

NOTES

✿ Stage 2 only: before cooking, add a sprinkle of ground cinnamon to the batter and mix.

Buckwheat Crepes GF P ✳ 🍎

SERVES 3; PREPARATION TIME 7 MINUTES, COOKING TIME 20 MINUTES

1 cup buckwheat flour (GF)

½ cup brown rice flour (GF)

½ teaspoon bicarbonate of soda (baking soda)

2 cups organic malt-free soy milk or rice milk (see 'Non-dairy milks', p. 77)

2 eggs, lightly beaten (or egg-free equivalent)

½ teaspoon real vanilla essence

rice bran oil, to coat the pan

rice malt syrup, to serve

2 medium bananas, sliced (A)

In a bowl, mix together both the flours and the bicarbonate of soda and sift if necessary. Gradually add the milk into the dry ingredients, mixing until lump-free. Mix in the eggs and vanilla essence.

Oil a small non-stick frying pan on medium–high heat. Pour in a thin layer of batter and cook lightly on each side, turning when the mixture begins to bubble. Repeat the process for each crepe. Top each crepe with rice malt syrup and sliced banana and fold them in half if desired.

Stewed Pear GF 🍎

MAKES 4 SERVES; PREPARATION TIME 5 MINUTES, COOKING TIME 5 MINUTES

4 large pears, peeled and sliced into thick wedges

filtered water, enough to cover

Place the pears and water in a medium-sized saucepan and boil for 3–5 minutes (don't cook for too long as the pears will go mushy). Remove from the heat, strain the liquid (you can keep this for drinking) and serve the pears.

NOTES

❉ For baby food, purée the stewed pears in a food processor or cook for longer and mash with a fork. You can freeze the leftovers, divided in an ice-cube tray, and defrost fresh each day.

❉ You can use puréed stewed pear to make icy poles for your child.

Pear Muffins ✳ ●P

MAKES 12 MUFFINS; PREPARATION TIME 15 MINUTES, COOKING TIME 15 MINUTES

1 egg (or egg-free substitute)
⅓ cup golden syrup (for eczema-safe sweeteners see p. 76; see Notes)
1 cup organic soy milk (G) or rice milk (see 'Non-dairy milks', p. 77)
½ teaspoon real vanilla essence
⅓ cup rice bran oil
2 cups spelt flour (G) (wholemeal if available)
3 teaspoons baking powder (wheat-free)
½ teaspoon bicarbonate of soda (baking soda)
2 large ripe pears, peeled and diced

Preheat the oven to 180°C (355°F). Place paper patty pans into the holes of a 12-cup muffin tray (or alternatively grease the muffin tray holes with rice bran oil). In a food processor, blend the egg, golden syrup, milk and vanilla essence until smooth. Then, while the motor is running, open the shute and slowly drizzle in the rice bran oil and blend well until smooth and creamy.

In a separate bowl, sift the flour, baking powder and bicarbonate of soda and mix. Add the dry ingredients to the wet ingredients and briefly mix on low speed until combined (or alternatively use a spoon to mix). Then using a spoon, gently mix in the diced pear. Spoon the mixture into each muffin cup, filling each only three-quarters. Bake for 15 minutes or until slightly golden on top. Test with a toothpick to see if cooked; the toothpick should come out clean.

NOTES

❋ These muffins can be stored in the freezer for 3 months.

❋ If golden syrup is not available use real maple syrup or rice malt syrup (rice malt syrup is not as sweet).

❋ If using egg, don't eat the raw muffin mixture (see 'Biotin', p. 96).

❋ Stage 2 only: if you are not sensitive to cinnamon, sprinkle a little cinnamon into the muffin mix before cooking.

New Anzac Cookies ✿

MAKES 20 BISCUITS; PREPARATION TIME 15 MINUTES, COOKING TIME 20 MINUTES

These sweet Anzac biscuits are butter- and dairy-free. Although this recipe is wheat-free it's not suitable if you have a wheat allergy or gluten intolerance.

1½ cups rolled oats (G)

1 cup plain spelt flour (G) (wholemeal if available)

⅔ cup fine raw sugar

½ cup rice bran oil

1 tablespoon golden syrup

½ teaspoon bicarbonate of soda (baking soda)

2 tablespoons water

Preheat the oven to 150°C (300°F). Line two baking trays with baking paper. In a mixing bowl, combine the oats, spelt flour and sugar.

In a small saucepan on high heat, combine the rice bran oil and golden syrup and cook until the syrup begins to bubble (stir the mixture continuously to ensure it does not burn). Promptly add the bicarbonate of soda and mix with a spoon until it foams. Quickly remove the saucepan from the heat before the syrup burns, and pour the hot foaming liquid onto the dry ingredients and mix well. Then add the water and mix until well combined.

The cookie dough should be wet and stick when pressed into shape. Make into 20 small balls (approx, 2cm/¾in wide) and place them on the trays (they will expand so allow room between them). Bake for 12–15 minutes or until golden brown.

Banana on Sticks GF 🍎

SERVES 4; PREPARATION TIME 5 MINUTES, ALLOW FOR FREEZING TIME

4 small ripe bananas, peeled (A)

4 iceblock (popsicle/ice lolly) sticks

Put the bananas on sticks by piercing them from one end to make them look like icy poles. Wrap each banana in plastic wrap and put them in the freezer overnight.

Recipes for natural cleaning products

Vinegar Cleaning Spray

Vinegar is naturally antibacterial and it cuts through grease, making it a good all-purpose cleaning spray for kitchen benchtops, toilets, baths and tabletops. Do not use vinegar on marble surfaces.

1 x empty spray bottle (see Notes)
equal parts water and white vinegar

Place the vinegar and water into the bottle and mix.

NOTES

✽ Cheap plastic spray bottles, bought from the discount shop, may buckle out of shape when vinegar is placed in it for prolonged periods. Recycle an old cleaning product spray bottle as these are generally made with stronger plastic.

Baking Soda Scrub

Bicarbonate of soda (baking soda), from the baking section in most supermarkets, makes a handy (and cheap) all-purpose scrub. Sprinkle some onto a damp cloth and use it to clean bathroom and kitchen surfaces. Along with a scrubbing brush, it's perfect for cleaning the bath.

Chapter 19
Eczema-safe food charts

The food charts on the following pages are designed to show you what foods to favour if you have eczema. To avoid confusion, the first time you look at the food charts, just notice the headings 'Strongly Alkalising', 'Alkalising', 'Acidifying' and 'Strongly Acidifying' and familiarise yourself with the foods in each column. The 'Strongly Alkalising' foods are the best ones for balancing the body's pH. Keep in mind that many of the 'Acidifying' foods, such as fish, beans and wholegrains, are an important part of a healthy diet so you do not need to avoid all of the acidifying foods, just the ones written in grey, which are not eczema-safe.

The next step when looking at the food charts is to note which foods are written in **bold** type. These are the foods you should favour during Stage 1 or while you suffer from eczema. As you can see in the charts, some of the best 'Strongly alkalising' foods (such as broccoli and dark leafy greens) are also rich in irritating chemicals so while they are very healthy foods, they are not eczema-safe (but they may be slowly introduced to the diet once your eczema has healed).

These charts are particularly useful if you've identified a food that causes your eczema to flare up. For example, if you react to beetroot you can look on the vegetable chart and you'll see it's marked with the letter **S**: this means it contains moderate salicylates and it can indicate you may be sensitive to salicylates. If this occurs, look at Table 4, 'Nutrients for liver detoxification' p. 49, and see which nutrients you need to take to help your liver process salicylates.

Symbols and abbreviations

bold Stage 1 eczema-safe ingredient to enjoy (allergy permitting)

grey ingredients to avoid while you have eczema

S moderate salicylate content

SS high to very high salicylate content

Su contains sulfites

A contains amines (or is histamine producing)

AA high to very high amine content

M natural flavour enhancer or artificial MSG

GI food with a high glycemic index (use chromium to balance blood sugar)

G contains gluten

? alkalising/acidifying status unconfirmed

! may cause severe reactions (avoid it!)

PS may contain preservatives and/or artificial sweetener/flavours/colours

Eczema-safe food charts: Stage 1

Condiments, sweeteners, sweets, salt and spices: Stage 1

Strongly alkalising	Alkalising	Acidifying	Strongly acidifying
apple cider vinegar (SS) (AA)(Su)	Celtic/macro sea salt, unrefined	barley malt	artificial sweetener (PS)(!)
	chives	carob powder	chewing gum and candy (SS)(PS)(!)
	cinnamon (SS)	hydrolysed vegetable protein (AA)(M)	chocolate (AA)(PS)
	garlic	jams (jellies) (SS)(Su)	golden syrup
	ginger (SS)	licorice (SS)	gravy (SS)(M)(AA)(Su)
	herbs, other (SS)	maple syrup, real	mayonnaise (SS)(AA) (PS)(!)
	lecithin granules, soy	molasses (S)	meat extracts (SS)(M)
	vanilla, whole bean	soy sauce (AA)(M)(G)	mustard (SS)(AA)
	rice malt syrup	stock cubes (SS)(M)(AA)	salt, table/processed (PS)
	saffron	tamari sauce (M)(AA)	sugar
	spices, all (SS)	vanilla essence, real	tomato paste, ketchup (SS)(M)(A)
	curry powder and curry paste (SS)(!)	honey (SS)	vinegar, other types (SS)(Su)

Beverages: Stage 1

Strongly alkalising	Alkalising	Acidifying	Strongly acidifying
broth, homemade	almond milk (AA)(SS)	beer (S)(A)(Su)	alcohol: wine (Su), brandy liqueur, port, rum, sherry (SS)(M)(AA)
green detox powder supplements (SS)(!)	herbal teas (not green tea) (SS)	fruit juice (SS)(Su)	
		green tea (SS)	
vegetable juice, fresh (SS)	**mineral water, non-carbonated, no flavour**	milk, dairy	black tea (SS)(Su)
Tarzan Juice	**water, plain filtered or from a spring**	mineral water, carbonated, no flavour	chocolate drinks (AA)(PS)
Healthy Skin Juice (S)	vegetable juice, packaged (SS)(M)(A)(Su)	**rice milk, plain and organic (GI)**	coffee (S)(PS)
liquid chlorophyll (SS)			cordial (SS)(PS)
		soy milk, plain and organic (G)	dried soup mixes (Su) (SS)(M)(PS)
		soy milk, organic and malt-free (GF)	soft drink (sodas) (SS)(PS)
		tomato juice and soup (SS)(M)(A)(Su)	tap water

Nuts, seeds, oils and fats: Stage 1

Strongly alkalising	Alkalising	Acidifying	Strongly acidifying
	almonds (SS)(AA)	canola oil (PS)	hazelnuts (SS)(AA)
	almond milk (AA)(SS)	**cashew nuts, raw, unsalted**	hydrogenated fats
	almond oil (S)		lard
	Brazil nuts (SS)	cashews, roasted (SS)(AA)	margarine (PS)
	butter, pure	coconut oil (SS)(AA)	peanuts (SS)(AA)
	cold-pressed 'extra virgin' oils (unheated)	cold-pressed 'extra-virgin' oils when heated	pecan nuts (SS)(AA)
	linseeds/flaxseeds (S)	pine nuts (SS)(AA)	pistachio nuts (SS)(AA)
	flaxseed oil (S)	poppyseed (?)	pumpkin seeds (SS)(AA)
	extra virgin olive oil (SS)(AA)	**rice bran oil (?)**	
		refined safflower oil (no antioxidant, not 'extra virgin')	sunflower seeds (SS)(AA)
		sesame seeds (SS)(AA)	walnuts (SS)(AA)

Vegetables: Stage 1

Strongly alkalising	Alkalising	Acidifying	Strongly acidifying
barley grass (G)(SS)(!)	artichoke (SS)	bamboo shoots	corn (SS)
beetroot, beets, raw (S)	asparagus (S)	peas (fresh or frozen) (S)(M)	gherkin, (SS)(AA)(Su)
broccoli (SS)(M)(A)	**brussels sprouts**	peas, dried and cooked	pickled vegetables (SS) (AA)(Su)
cucumber (SS)	**cabbage, white and red**	silverbeet, cooked (SS)(M)(AA)	
dark leafy greens, raw (SS)	**carrot (S)**		
kale, raw (SS)	capsicum (pepper) (SS)		
rocket (arugula) (SS)	cauliflower (SS)		
spinach, raw (SS)(M)(A)	**celery**		
alfalfa sprouts (SS)	chicory (S)		
lentil sprouts	Chinese greens (S)		
mung bean sprouts	**choko (chayote)**		
snow pea (mangetout) sprouts (S)	eggplant (aubergine) (SS)(AA)		
watercress (SS)	endive (S)		
wheatgrass juice (SS)(!)	**green beans**		
	leek		
	cos lettuce (romaine) (S)		
	lettuce, iceberg		
	marrow (S)		
	mushroom (SS)(M)(AA)		
	olive (SS)(AA)		
	onion (SS)		
	parsnip (S)(GI)		
	pumpkin (winter squash) (S)(GI)		
	radish (SS)		
	snow pea (mangetout) (S)		
	spring onion (shallot/scallion)		
	swede (rutabaga)		
	baby (pattypan) squash (S)		
	turnip (S)		
	yam (S)		
	zucchini (courgette) (S)		

Potatoes are listed on the carbohydrate table, p. 257.

Fruit, fresh and dried: Stage 1

Strongly alkalising	Alkalising	Acidifying	Strongly acidifying
grapefruit (SS)(AA)	apricot, dried (SS)(Su)	apples (SS)	blackcurrant (SS)
lemon (SS)(AA)	avocado (SS)(AA)	apricot, raw (SS)	blackthorn berry (SS)
lime (SS)(AA)	banana, sugar variety (SS)(AA)	berries, most varieties (SS)	kiwi fruit (SS)(AA)
	banana, other (A)	cherry (SS)	mandarin (SS)(AA)
	date, dried (SS)(AA)(GI)	coconut (SS)(AA)	orange (SS)(AA)
	raisins (SS)(M)(AA)	dried fruits (SS)(Su)	mulberry (SS)
	tomato, raw (SS)(M)(AA)	figs (SS)(AA)(Su)	nectarine (SS)
		grape (SS)(M)(AA)	pineapple (SS)(AA)
		mango (S)	
		papaya (A)	
		pawpaw (A)	
		pear, peeled	
		persimmon (S)	
		plum (SS)(M)(AA)	
		pomegranate (SS)	
		prune (SS)(M)(AA)	
		raspberry (SS)(AA)	
		strawberry (SS)	
		tomato, cooked (SS)(M)(AA)	
		watermelon (SS)(GI)	

Note: Coconut products such as fresh coconut, coconut oil and coconut milk are very rich in salicylates (SS) and amines (AA) so they should be avoided during Stage 1 of the Eczema Diet.

Carbohydrates — potatoes, grains, flours, breads: Stage 1

Strongly alkalising	Alkalising	Acidifying	Strongly acidifying
	potato, carisma (best choice)	amaranth (GI)(!)	basmati rice
	potato, new (S)	baby rice cereal, plain	corn (SS)
	potato, white	barley (G)	corn cakes (corn crackers) (SS)
	sweet potato (S)	brown rice (GI)	corn chips, tacos (S)
	sprouted grains	buckwheat	cornflakes (SS)(GI)
		buckwheat pasta (no wheat)	cornflour (GI)
		cous cous (semolina, durum wheat) (G)	millet (GI)
		cracked wheat (G)	pasta, gluten-free (caution: corn/maize)
		muesli (granola) (SS)(A)	pasta, white, wheat (G)
		oats, rolled (G)	polenta (cornmeal) (SS)(GI)
		oat milk (no honey) (G)(GI)	processed wheat cereals (GI)(G)
		quinoa (GI)	rice crackers, plain (GI)
		rice milk, plain with sunflower oil (GI)	white rice, jasmine rice (GI)
		pumpernickel	white bread (GI)(G)
		rye flour (G)	flour, white (GI)(G)
		soy flour (?)	yeast breads (G)
		sago, tapioca (GI)(?)	
		spelt pasta (G)	
		spelt bread (G)	
		wholegrain wheat bread (G)	

Protein — legumes, dairy, milk, fish, poultry and meat: Stage 1

Strongly alkalising	Alkalising	Acidifying	Strongly acidifying
	butter, pure and unheated	anchovy (AA)	beef
	buttermilk, fresh	**beans, most (not broad bean)**	butter, heated
	egg yolk	broad bean (SS)	cheese (AA)
	ghee/clarified butter	**chicken**	fish, pickled or smoked (AA)
	whey, fresh	**fish, fresh (see p. 71)**	ice-cream (PS)
		chickpeas (garbanzo beans)	kefir
		lamb, lean	lobster
		lentils	meat pies (SS)(M)(AA)
		milk, dairy	peanut (SS)(AA)
		yoghurt, plain and organic	pork, ham, bacon (AA)
		soy milk, organic	processed deli meats (SS)(M)(AA)
		tempeh (AA)(M)	**salmon (AA)**
		tuna, canned in olive oil (SS)(AA)	sausages (SS)(M)(A)
		tuna, canned in springwater (AA)	yoghurt, sweetened, fruit (SS)
		veal	

Chapter 20

Eczema-safe shopping guides

The first shopping guide, for Stage 1, lists the main food products to buy while you have eczema, and the Stage 2 guide, ideally, should be used after your eczema clears up. Brand suggestions are included to make shopping easier but other brands can also be suitable, just check the ingredients before purchase. If the brands mentioned are not available in your area, you may find you need to do some experimenting to find the products that suit you. For example, the flavour, texture and general suitability of gluten-free products, such as pasta, can vary considerably between brands, so if you don't like one or find your skin isn't improving as it should on the diet, please persevere and try others until you discover the ones that work for you.

Please note the shopping lists do not account for age and feeding ability and not all ingredients are suitable for small children or those with gluten intolerance (or less common allergies such as rice allergy). Also, the shopping lists include ingredients that are not in the Eczema Diet recipes, so you have the option to use them to make your own recipes. This can be useful if you have food allergies to some of the foods in Stage 1 and you need alternatives to increase variety in your diet.

Eczema-safe shopping guide: Stage 1

Fruit

- [ ] bananas (not sugar variety)
- [ ] pears
- [ ] papaya or pawpaw

Veg + herb

- [ ] parsley
- [ ] garlic (not Chinese)
- [ ] brussels sprouts
- [ ] chives (not in recipes)
- [ ] choko (chayote) (not in recipes)
- [ ] leeks
- [ ] iceberg lettuce
- [ ] cos (romaine) lettuce
- [ ] mung bean sprouts (fresh only/check use-by date)
- [ ] celery
- [ ] cabbage, red or white
- [ ] green beans
- [ ] spring onions/shallots (scallions)
- [ ] potatoes e.g. carisma, new (not desiree, sebago, pontiac, nardine)
- [ ] sweet potato
- [ ] carrots
- [ ] swede (rutabaga)
- [ ] beetroot, fresh not canned

Health food

- [ ] flaxseed oil, only buy if refrigerated (e.g. Melrose organic flaxseed oil)
- [ ] linseeds/flaxseeds, whole (not pre-ground, not LSA)
- [ ] soy lecithin granules (e.g. Nature First or Soland)

Non-dairy milk + drinks

- [ ] organic soy milk, favour refrigerated over long-life tetra packs and 'organic whole soybean' (not soy isolate, no flavourings)
- [ ] malt-free soy milk
- [ ] organic rice milk
- [ ] oat milk (optional, not in recipes)
- [ ] water filter jug (e.g. Brita)

Oil

- [ ] rice bran oil

Grains, breads + cereals

- [ ] spelt sourdough bread, preservative-free (e.g. Sonoma spelt sourdough)
- [ ] gluten-free bread, if necessary (preservative-free; check ingredients)
- [ ] basmati rice (not jasmine or other white rice)
- [ ] brown rice (low GI if available)
- [ ] barley
- [ ] buckwheat, roasted (not in recipes)
- [ ] buckwheat pasta (wheat-free)
- [ ] gluten-free pasta (preferably maize/corn-free)
- [ ] rolled oats (wheat-free if possible)
- [ ] puffed brown rice cereal, plain (not in recipes)
- [ ] quinoa grains (not puffed)

Sweeteners + flavourings

- [ ] rice malt syrup (e.g. Pureharvest)
- [ ] real maple syrup (optional)
- [ ] golden syrup (if baking)
- [ ] vanilla bean or real vanilla essence
- [ ] carob powder (not cocoa powder)

Baking + flours

- [ ] spelt flour (wholemeal, if available)
- [ ] gluten-free self-raising flour (e.g. White Wings Gluten Free)
- [ ] buckwheat flour
- [ ] rice flour (brown, if available)
- [ ] egg replacer (e.g. Orgran No Egg)
- [ ] bicarbonate of soda (baking soda) (for baking)
- [ ] baking powder (for baking; not in recipes)

☐ citric acid (flavour/lemon replacer), baking section

☐ arrowroot flour (not in recipes)

☐ soy flour (not in recipes)

☐ rye flour (not in recipes)

Grain crackers + biscuits

☐ rye crispbread, wholemeal (no wheat) (e.g. Multigrain Ryvitas®)

☐ wholegrain or plain rice crackers, no flavour enhancer (e.g. Sakata™)

☐ wholegrain plain rice cakes (no flavour enhancer or corn/maize)

Meat, fish + other refrigerated

Note: do not buy all items on the same day

☐ free range/organic chicken, antibiotic-free (thigh fillets, breast or whole for roast)

☐ 1 large or 2 small chicken carcasses (for Therapeutic Broth recipe)

☐ 2 large beef bones with a little meat on them (for Therapeutic Broth recipe)

☐ lean veal, e.g. veal steaks (not pre-crumbed; not in recipes)

☐ Frenched lamb cutlets or lean lamb, fat trimmed

☐ turkey, uncooked or organic (not deli meats, no flavour enhancer; not in recipes)

☐ trout, rainbow trout (not frozen or preserved/packaged)

☐ flathead or small white fish (not basa, snapper, swordfish, marlin, flake/shark, ling, perch, gemfish, large barramundi or tuna)

☐ canned tuna, quality/chunky, in springwater or brine, (not oil or olive oil)

☐ canned salmon, in springwater or brine (no flavourings or oil)

Cans, jars + packets

☐ dried red lentils

☐ cashew nuts, raw, unsalted

☐ Celtic sea salt or macro sea salt

☐ dried beans (kidney, cannellini etc. not broad beans)

☐ canned beans

☐ dried split peas (not in recipes)

☐ soy beans, fresh or dried (not in recipes)

☐ chickpeas (garbanzo beans), dried or canned

☐ dried parsley flakes

☐ dried garlic powder, no additives (not garlic salt)

Additives to avoid

colours* 102, 104, 107, 110, 122–129, 132, 133, 142, 151, 155; 160b annatto 'natural colour' (160a is okay); preservatives 200–203, 210–213, 220–228, 249–252, 280–283 (bread: 282 calcium propionate); antioxidant 310–321; flavour enhancer/MSG 620–635; 'natural flavour' can be MSG; artificial sweetener 951/aspartame, 954; (*American: blue 1 and 2; green 3; red 2, 3, 4 and 40; yellow 5 and 6)

Eczema-safe shopping guide: Stage 2

Note: Stage 2 foods are highlighted in **bold**.

Fruit

- [ ] bananas
- [ ] pears
- [ ] papaya or pawpaw
- [ ] **golden delicious apples**
- [ ] **red delicious apples**
- [ ] **blueberries**
- [ ] **watermelon**
- [ ] **lemon or lime**

Veg + herb

- [ ] parsley
- [ ] garlic (not Chinese)
- [ ] brussels sprouts
- [ ] chives (not in recipes)
- [ ] choko (chayote) (not in recipes)
- [ ] leeks
- [ ] iceberg lettuce
- [ ] cos (romaine) lettuce
- [ ] mung bean sprouts
- [ ] celery
- [ ] cabbage, red or white
- [ ] green beans
- [ ] spring onions/shallots (scallions)
- [ ] potatoes, e.g. carisma, new (not desiree, sebago, pontiac, nardine)
- [ ] sweet potato
- [ ] carrots
- [ ] swedes (rutabaga)
- [ ] beetroot, fresh not canned
- [ ] snow peas (mangetout)
- [ ] **snow pea (mangetout) sprouts**
- [ ] **asparagus**
- [ ] **chicory**
- [ ] **endive**
- [ ] **bok choy (pak choy)**
- [ ] **mint**
- [ ] **basil**
- [ ] **coriander (cilantro)**
- [ ] **onion, red or white**
- [ ] **baby (pattypan) squash**
- [ ] **turnip**
- [ ] **yam**
- [ ] **green peas**

Health food

- [ ] flaxseed oil (must be refrigerated, preferably organic)
- [ ] linseeds/flaxseeds, whole
- [ ] soy lecithin granules
- [ ] **apple cider vinegar** (organic, not 'double strength')

Sweeteners + flavourings

- [ ] rice malt syrup
- [ ] real maple syrup (optional)
- [ ] golden syrup (if baking)
- [ ] vanilla bean or real vanilla essence
- [ ] carob powder (not cocoa powder)

Non-dairy milks + drinks

- [ ] organic soy milk
- [ ] malt-free soy milk
- [ ] organic rice milk
- [ ] oat milk

Oil

- [ ] rice bran oil

Grains, breads + cereals

- [ ] spelt sourdough bread, preservative-free
- [ ] gluten-free bread, if necessary (preservative-free)
- [ ] basmati rice
- [ ] brown rice (low GI if available)
- [ ] barley
- [ ] buckwheat, roasted (not in recipes)
- [ ] buckwheat pasta (wheat-free)
- [ ] gluten-free pasta
- [ ] rolled oats (wheat-free if possible)
- [ ] puffed brown rice cereal, plain
- [ ] quinoa grains (not puffed)

Baking + flours

- [ ] spelt flour
- [ ] gluten-free self-raising flour
- [ ] buckwheat flour
- [ ] rice flour (preferably brown)
- [ ] egg replacer/substitute
- [ ] bicarbonate of soda (baking soda) (for baking)
- [ ] baking powder (for baking)
- [ ] citric acid (flavour/lemon replacer)
- [ ] arrowroot flour (not in recipes)
- [ ] soy flour (not in recipes)
- [ ] rye flour (not in recipes)

Grain crackers + biscuits

- [ ] rye crispbread, wholemeal (no wheat)
- [ ] wholegrain or plain rice crackers, no flavour enhancer
- [ ] wholegrain plain rice cakes, no flavour enhancer, no corn/maize

Meat, fish + other refrigerated

Note: do not buy all items on the same day

- [ ] free range/organic chicken, antibiotic-free (thigh fillets, breast or whole for roast)
- [ ] 2 chicken carcasses (for Therapeutic Broth recipe) or chicken necks, lamb/beef bones
- [ ] lean veal, e.g. veal steaks (not pre-crumbed)
- [ ] lean lamb (not shanks/cheap mince etc.)
- [ ] turkey, uncooked or organic (not deli meats/flavour enhancer)
- [ ] trout, rainbow trout (**or salmon**) (not frozen or preserved/packaged)
- [ ] flathead or smaller-sized fish (not basa, snapper, swordfish, marlin, flake/shark, perch, gemfish, large barramundi or tuna)

- [ ] canned tuna, quality/chunky, in springwater or brine, (not oil or olive oil)
- [ ] canned salmon, in springwater or brine (no flavourings or oil)
- [ ] **V&Vn: firm tofu**, plain/unflavoured (optional, not tempeh or vegan patties)
- [ ] **free-range eggs** or egg replacer
- [ ] **pure organic butter** (allergy permitting, no additives or oils)

Cans, jars + packets

- [ ] dried red lentils
- [ ] canned brown lentils
- [ ] cashew nuts, raw, unsalted
- [ ] Celtic sea salt or macro sea salt or iodised sea salt (no anti-caking agent)
- [ ] dried beans (kidney, cannellini etc. not broad beans)
- [ ] canned beans, no flavourings
- [ ] dried split peas (green or yellow)
- [ ] soybeans, fresh or dried (not in recipes)
- [ ] chickpeas (garbanzo beans), dried or canned
- [ ] dried parsley flakes
- [ ] dried garlic powder, no additives (not garlic salt)
- [ ] **organic tomato sauce (ketchup)**
- [ ] **bamboo shoots (not in recipes)**
- [ ] **cinnamon**
- [ ] **ground cumin**

Additives to avoid

colours* 102, 104, 107, 110, 122–129, 132, 133, 142, 151, 155; 160b annatto 'natural colour' (160a is okay); preservatives 200–203, 210–213, 220–228, 249–252, 280–283 (bread: 282 calcium propionate); antioxidant 310–321; flavour enhancer/MSG 620–635; 'natural flavour' can be MSG; artificial sweetener 951/aspartame, 954; (*American: blue 1 and 2; green 3; red 2, 3, 4 and 40; yellow 5 and 6)

Diet diary

You can photocopy the diet diary below and record what you eat each day to help you identify the cause of any adverse reactions. You can also rate how your skin looks at the end of each day, where it says 'Rate your eczema', and make notes on any adverse reactions. Rate your skin from 1 to 10: a score of 1 means your eczema is at its worst or covering a large part of your body, a score of 10 means you are eczema-free, and so on.

Day___	Breakfast	Morning snack	Lunch	Afternoon snack	Dinner	Rate your eczema /10

Day___	Breakfast	Morning snack	Lunch	Afternoon snack	Dinner	Rate your eczema /10

Resources

Eczema supplements

Karen Fischer's websites

www.beautyby.com.au

www.theeczemadiet.com

Skin care information or support

Eczema Association of Australasia
(Australia)

Phone: 1300 300 182

www.eczema.org.au

National Eczema Association (USA)

Phone: 415-499-3474 or 800-818-7546

www.nationaleczema.org

National Eczema Society (UK)

Helpline: 0800 089 1122

www.eczema.org

Eczema Scotland

www.eczemascotland.org

European Federation of Allergy and
Airways Diseases Patients Association
(EFA)

www.efanet.org

Itchy Kids (New Zealand)

www.itchykids.org.nz

Feeding fussy children

Inspire your fussy child to love healthy
food and ask for more …

Healthy Family, Happy Family, Karen
Fischer (Exisle Publishing)

www.exislepublishing.com

Allergy tests

Ask your doctor for a referral for allergy
testing in your area.

Liver detoxification function test

HealthScope Pathology (Melbourne,
Australia)

Test: Functional Liver Detoxification
Profile (salicylate/chemical sensitivity
test) Phone: 1300 554 480 (within
Australia)

www.healthscopepathology.com.au

Breathing exercises for stress management

Breathe For Life, Sophie Gabriel

www.breatheforlife.com

sophie@breatheforlife.com

Carisma potato information

www.theeczemadiet.com

Acknowledgments

I have many people to thank for their input during the creation of the Eczema Diet. Firstly, my daughter was the inspiration for this research and she helped design two of the dessert recipes. My children, Ayva and Jack, are the first people to test my recipes and they have helped me to grow in so many ways so I dedicate this book to both of them.

Over the years, my patients and readers have inspired me to continue researching eczema. In particular, a boy called Jacob whose mother wrote to me months after their initial consultation to tell me of the pain and embarrassment Jacob had suffered while he had eczema and how happy they both felt when Jacob's skin healed. The before and after photos of Jacob brought tears to my eyes and I resolved to continue with my work. I really appreciate the feedback from my former patients and I admire their dedication to follow the diet and improve their skin (and on occasion, tell me straight what's working and what isn't!). Thank you all for your feedback, especially Mary Washington, Amanda Essex, Linda Balfour, Natalya L., Bianca Rothwell, Anandhi Krishnakumar, Claudine Hardy, Meaghan Ottewill, Karma Montagne, Bronwyn Air, Jenny Bangor, Lyn McPherson, Cathi Firth and Anna Kluge. And thanks to Bianca Rothwell for forwarding a couple of her recipes so I could pass them on to other eczema sufferers.

My mother is my greatest support and I owe her a mountain of gratitude for her advice, love and encouragement, and my dad, for his interest in health — both of you have provided me with a strong foundation to persevere in my field of work, which I adore.

I really appreciate the words of support from Professor Gary Leong, director of KOALA Healthy Life Clinic at the Mater Children's Hospital — thank you for your testimonials and encouragement over the past three years.

I want to thank Professor Michael J. Cork, Head of Academic Unit of Dermatology Research and Les Hunter from The University of Sheffield, who kindly supplied the 'brick wall model of the skin' diagram on p. 12. The liver detoxification data obtained from HealthScope Pathology in Melbourne, and the scientific research on eczema, allergies, nutrients and food intolerance were instrumental in creating and refining this program, so I'd like to thank all scientists and medical researchers for publishing their valuable work. The Eczema Association of Australasia does a wonderful job supporting eczema sufferers and I'm grateful for their newsletters, support and online information.

I'd like to say a heartfelt thank you to Selwa Anthony for believing in my writing and to Benny St John Thomas and the team at Exisle Publishing for publishing my books and for making them look beautiful. A special thank you goes to my editors Anouska Jones and Karen Gee: I feel so blessed to have editors who understand health and they enhance my work in so many ways.

This has been a long process and I'm sure my eczema research will continue. I wish I could have supplied more recipes in this book but the present ones took me ten years to design and refine. To increase variety, I encourage you to experiment with the eczema-safe ingredients and design additional recipes for yourself, and if you'd like to see your eczema-safe recipes (and your name) in the next book you can submit your recipes for review via my website. Thank you for reading my books and for entrusting me with your health. May your eczema heal swiftly.

Warm wishes,
Karen

Endnotes

Introduction

1. Palmer, C.N.A. et al., 2006, 'Common loss-of-function variants of the epidermal barrier protein filaggrin are a major predisposing factor for atopic dermatitis', *Nature Genetics*, vol. 38, no. 4, pp. 441–6.
2. Ordovas, J.M. and Corella, D., 2004, 'Nutritional Genomics', *Annual Reviews of Genomics and Human Genetics*, vol. 5, pp. 71–118.

Chapter 1

1. Brenninkmeijer, E.E.A., et al., 2008, 'Diagnostic criteria for atopic dermatitis: a systematic review', *British Journal of Dermatology*, vol. 158, pp. 754–65.
2. Cork, M.J. et al., 'New understanding to the predisposition of atopic eczema and sensitive skin', retrieved 1 May 2011: www.allergyuk.org
3. ibid.
4. Cork, M.J., et al., 2006, 'New perspectives on epidermal barrier dysfunction in atopic dermatitis: gene-environment interactions', *Journal of Allergy and Clinical Immunology*, vol 118, pp. 3–21.
5. Reitamo, S., Luger, T.A. and Steinhoff, M. (eds), 2008, *Textbook of Atopic Dermatitis*, Informa Healthcare, London.
6. Rich, A.C., 13 May 1882, 'On the treatment of eczema by diet', *British Medical Journal*, pp. 695–6.

Chapter 2

1. Su, J., 2006, 'The skin barrier Q&A with dermatologist Dr John Su, Royal Children's Hospital Melbourne', *Eczema Association of Australasia*, retrieved 12 August 2010: http://www.eczema.org.au/
2. Palmer, C.N.A., et al., 2006, loc. cit.
3. ibid.
4. Cordain, L., et al., 2005, 'Origins and evolution of the western diet: health implications for the 21st century', *American Journal of Clinical Nutrition*, vol. 81, pp. 341–54.
5. Sure, B. and Ford, Z.W., 1942, 'The influence of thiamine, riboflavin, pyridoxine and pantothenic acid deficiencies on nitrogen metabolism', *Journal of Nutrition*, vol. 24, no. 5, pp. 405–26.
6. Cordain, L., et al., 2005, loc. cit.
7. Cordain. L. 2005, 'Implications for the role of diet in acne', *Seminars in Cutaneous Medicine and Surgery*, vol. 24, no. 2, reprinted in *Rosacea News*, 'Could rosacea be caused by diet?'
8. Cordain, L., et al., 2005, loc. cit.
9. Cordain, L. et al., 2002, '*Acne vulgaris*, a disease of western civilisation', *Archives of Dermatology*, vol. 138, no. 12, pp. 1584–90.
10. Cordain. L. 2005, loc. cit.
11. Ordovas, J.M. and Corella, D., loc. cit.
12. Heinrich, J., et al., 2001, 'Allergic sensitization and diet: ecological analysis in selected European cities', *European Respiratory Journal*, vol. 17, no. 3, pp. 395–402.
13. Hix, L. et al., 2004, 'Bioactive carotenoids: potent antioxidants and regulators of gene expression', *Redox Report*, vol. 9, no. 4, pp. 181–91.
14. Do, R., et al., 2011, 'The effect of chromosome 9p21 variants on

cardiovascular disease may be modified by dietary intake: evidence from a case/control and a prospective study', *PLoS Medicine*, vol. 9, no. 10, retrieved 20 October 2011: http://www.plosmedicine.org.

15. Sampson, H.A. and Jolie, P.L., 1984, 'Increased plasma histamine concentrations after food challenges in children with atopic dermatitis', *New England Journal of Medicine*, vol. 311, pp. 372–6.

16. Sicherer, S.H. et al., 1999, 'Food hyper-sensitivity and atopic dermatitis: pathophysiology, epidemiology, diagnosis and management', *Journal of Allergy & Clinical Immunology*, vol. 104, no. 3, pp. S114–22.

17. Maintz, L. and Novak, N., 2007, 'Histamine and histamine intolerance', *American Journal of Clinical Nutrition*, vol. 85, no. 5, pp. 1185–96.

18. Sicherer, S.H. et al., loc. cit.

19. Reitamo, S., et al. 2008, 'Possible clinical associations of atopic dermatitis with bronchial asthma', *Textbook of Atopic Dermatitis*, Chapter 8, Reitamo, S., Luger, T.A. and Steinhoff, M. (eds), Informa Healthcare, London.

20. Warner J.O., 2001, ETAC Study Group, 'Early treatment of atopic child. A double-blinded, randomized, placebo-controlled trial of cetirizine in preventing the onset of asthma in children with atopic dermatitis: 18 months' treatment and 18 months' post-treatment follow-up', *Journal of Allergy & Clinical Immunology*, vol. 108, pp. 929–37.

21. Worm, M., et al., 2009, 'Exogenous histamine aggravates eczema in a subgroup of patients with atopic dermatitis', *Acta Dermato-Venereologica*, vol. 89, pp 52–6.

22. Maintz, L. et al., 2006, 'Evidence for a reduced histamine degradation capacity in a subgroup of patients with atopic eczema', *Journal of Allergy & Clinical Immunology*, vol. 117, no. 5, pp. 1106–12.

23. Ionescu, G.J., 2009, 'New insights in the pathogenesis of atopic disease', *Journal of Medicine and Life*, vol. 2, no. 2, pp. 145–54.

24. Loblay, R.H. and Swain, A.R., 2006, 'Food intolerance', *Recent Advances in Clinical Nutrition*, University of Sydney, RPA Hospital.

25. Maintz, L. and Novak, N., loc. cit.

26. Ionescu, G.J., loc. cit.

27. Maintz, L. and Novak, N., loc. cit.

28. ibid.

29. Johnston, C.S., et al., 1992, 'Antihistamine effect of supplemental ascorbic acid and neutrophil chemotaxis', *Journal of the American College of Nutrition*, vol. 11, no. 2, pp. 172–6.

30. Kahraman, A., et al., 2003, 'The antioxidative and antihistaminic properties of quercetin in ethanol-induced gastric lesions', *Toxicology*, vol. 183, no. 1–3, pp. 133–42.

31. DeMeo, M.T., et al., 2002, 'Intestinal permeation and gastrointestinal disease', *Journal of Clinical Gastroenterology*, ol. 34, no. 4, pp. 385–96.

32. Caffarelli, C., et al., 1998, 'Gastrointestinal symptoms in atopic eczema', *Archives of Disease in Childhood*, vol. 78, pp. 230–4.

33. ibid.

34. Pike, M.G., et al., 1986, 'Increased intestinal permeability in atopic eczema', *Journal of Investigative Dermatology*, vol. 86, pp. 101–4.

35. Jackson, P.G., et al., 1981, 'Intestinal permeability in patients with eczema and food allergy', *Lancet*, vol. 1, no. 8233, pp. 1285–6.

36. ibid.
37. Kahraman, A., et al., loc. cit.
38. DeMeo, loc. cit.
39. Kahraman, A., et al., loc. cit.
40. Randolf, B.S. et al., 2008, 'Atopic dermatitis: the role of fungi', *Textbook of Atopic Dermatitis*, Chapter 7, Reitamo, S., Luger, T.A. & Steinhoff, M. (eds), Informa Healthcare, London.
41. Beare, J.M., 1968, 'The association between *Candida albicans* and lesions of seborrhoeic eczema', *British Journal of Dermatology*, vol. 80, no. 10, pp. 675–81.
42. Randolf, B.S., et al., loc. cit.
43. Savolainen, J., et al., 1993, '*Candida albicans* and atopic dermatitis', *Clinical & Experimental Allergy*, vol. 23, no. 4, pp. 332–9.
44. Penders, J., et al., 2007, 'Gut microbiota composition and development of atopic manifestations in infancy: the KOALA Birth Cohort Study', *GUT*, vol. 56, no. 5, pp. 661–7.
45. Manku, M.S., 1984, 'Essential fatty acids in the plasma phospholipids of patients with atopic eczema', *British Journal of Dermatology*, vol. 110, pp. 643–8.
46. Horrobin, D.F., 2000, 'Essential fatty acid metabolism and its modification in atopic eczema', *American Journal of Clinical Nutrition*, vol. 71, no. 1, pp. S367–72.
47. Galli, E., et al., 1994, 'Analysis of polyunsaturated fatty acids in newborn sera: a screening tool for atopic disease?' *British Journal of Dermatology*, vol. 130, pp. 752–6.
48. Horrobin, D.F., loc. cit.
49. Sausenthaler, S. et al., 2006, 'Margarine and butter consumption, eczema and allergic sensitization in children', *Pediatric Allergy and Immunology*, vol. 17, no. 2, pp. 85–93.
50. Bolte, G, et al., 2001, 'Margarine consumption and allergy in children',
51. Sausenthaler, S., et al., 2007, 'Maternal diet during pregnancy in relation to eczema and allergic sensitization in the offspring at 2 years of age', *American Journal of Clinical Nutrition*, vol. 85, pp. 530–7.
52. Loblay, R.H. and Swain, A.R., 2006, 'Food Intolerance', *Recent Advances in Clinical Nutrition*, retrieved 1 April 2011: www.nsw.gov.au.
53. ibid.
54. Loblay, R.H. and Swain, A.R., loc. cit.
55. Gutman, A.B., Yu, T.F. and Sirota, J.H., 1955, 'A study by simultaneous clearance techniques of salicylate excretion in man. Effect of alkalinization of the urine by bicarbonate administration; effect of probenecid', *Journal of Clinical Investigation*, vol. 34, no. 5, pp. 711–21.
56. Garc Roché, M.O., 2006, 'Effect of ascorbic acid on the hepatotoxicity due to the daily intake of nitrate, nitrite and dimethylamine', *Food/ Nahrung*, vol. 31, no. 2, pp. 99–104.
57. Honikel, K.O., 2008, 'The use and control of nitrate and nitrite for the processing of meat products', *Meat Science*, retrieved 16 April 2011: www.sciencedirect.com
58. Fiddler, W., et al., 1978, 'Inhibition of formation of volatile nitrosamines in fried bacon by the use of cure-solubilized α-tocopherol', *Journal of Agriculture and Food Chemistry*, vol. 26, no. 3, pp. 653–6.
59. Fiddler, W., et al., 1998, 'Nitrosamine formation in processed hams as related to reformulated elastic rubber netting', *Journal of Food Science*, vol. 63, pp. 276–8.
60. Honikel, K.O., 2008, loc. cit.
61. Loblay, R.H. and Swain, A.R., 2006, loc. cit.

American Journal of Respiratory and Critical Care Medicine, vol. 163, pp. 277–9.

62. Gupta, C., et al., 2010, 'Antioxidant and antimutagenic effect of quercetin against DEN induced hepatotoxicity in rat', *Phytotherapy Research*, vol. 24, no. 1, pp. 119–28.

63. Garc Roché, M.O., 2006, loc. cit.

64. Jerome, J.J. et al. 1976, 'Inhibition of amine-nitrite hepatotoxicity by α-toco-pherol', *Toxicology and Applied Pharmacology*, vol. 41, no. 3, pp. 575–83.

65. Loblay, R.H. and Swain, A.R., 2006, loc. cit.

66. McCann, D., et al., 2007, 'Food additives and hyperactive behaviour in 3-year-old and 8/9-year-old children in the community: a randomised, double-blinded, placebo-controlled trial', *The Lancet*, vol. 370, pp. 1560–7.

67. Dengate, S., 'Annato (160b)', Food Intolerance Network fact sheet: http://www.fedup.com.au/factsheets/additive-and-natural-chemical-factsheets/160b-annatto/.

68. Loblay, R.H. and Swain, A.R., 2006, loc. cit.

69. Dengate, S., 2009, 'Sulphites (220–228)', Food Intolerance Network fact sheet: http://www.fedup.com.au/factsheets/additive-and-natural-chemical-factsheets/220-228-sulphite-preservatives/.

70. Onyema, O.O., et al., 2006, 'Effect of vitamin E on monosodium glutamate induced hepatotoxicity and oxidative stress in rats', *Indian Journal of Biochemistry and Biophysics*, vol. 43, pp. 20–4.

71. Nakanishi, Y., et al, 2008, 'Monosodium glutamate (MSG): a villain and promoter of liver inflammation and dysplasia', *Journal of Autoimmunity*, vol. 30, no. 1–2, pp. 42–50.

72. Onyema, O.O., et al., loc. cit.

73. Uenishi, T., Sugiura, H. and Uehara, M., 2003, 'Role of foods in irregular aggravation of atopic dermatitis', *Journal of Dermatology*, vol. 30, pp. 91–7.

74. Rudzeviciene, O., et al., 2004, 'Lactose malabsorption in young Lithuanian children with atopic dermatitis', *Acta Paediatrica*, vol. 93, no. 4, pp. 482–6.

75. Loblay, R.H. & Swain, A.R., 2006, loc. cit.

Chapter 3

1. Smith, R.L. and Williams, R.T., 1970, 'History of the discovery of the conjugation mechanisms', pp. 1–19, *Metabolic Conjugation and Metabolic Hydrolysis*, Fishman, W.H. (ed.), Academic Press, New York.

2. Liska, D.J., 1998, 'The detoxification enzyme systems', *Alternative Medicine Review*, vol. 3, no. 3, pp. 187–98.

3. Minich, D.M. and Bland, J.S., 2007, 'Acid–alkaline balance: role in chronic disease and detoxification', *Alternative Therapies*, vol. 13, no. 4, pp. 62–5.

4. Manz, F., 2001, 'History of nutrition and acid-base physiology', *European Journal of Nutrition*, vol. 40, pp. 189–99.

5. Minich, D.M. and Bland, J.S., loc. cit.

6. Proudfoot, A.T., et al., 2004, 'Position paper on urine alkalinization', *Clinical Toxicology*, vol. 42, no. 1, pp. 1–26.

7. O'Malley, G.F., 2007, 'Emergency department management of the salicylate-poisoned patient', *Emergency Medicine Clinics of North America*, vol. 25, pp. 333–46.

8. Gutman, A.B., Yu, T.F. and Sirota, J.H., 1955, loc. cit.

9. Kurtz, I., et al., 1983, 'Effect of diet on plasma acid-base composition in normal humans', *Kidney International*, vol. 24, pp. 670–80.

10. Cordain, L., et al., 2005, 'Origins

and evolution of the western diet: health implications for the 21st century', *American Journal of Clinical Nutrition*, vol. 81, pp. 341–54.

11. Frassetto, L.A. et al., 1998, 'Estimation of net endogenous noncarbonic acid production in humans from diet potassium and protein contents', *American Journal of Clinical Nutrition*, vol. 68, pp. 576–83.

12. Sebastian, A. et al., 2002, 'Estimation of the net acid load of the diet of ancestral preagricultural *Homo sapiens* and their hominid ancestors', *American Journal of Clinical Nutrition*, vol. 76, pp. 1308–16.

13. Minich, D.M. and Bland, J.S., loc. cit.

14. Frassetto, L.A. et al., loc. cit.

15. New, S.A., 2001, 'Fruit and vegetable consumption and skeletal health: is there a positive link?' *Nutrition Bulletin*, vol. 26, no. 2, pp. 121–5.

Chapter 5

1. Hix et al., loc. cit.

2. Sausenthaler, S., et al., 2006, loc. cit.

3. Sausenthaler, S., et al., 2007, loc. cit.

Chapter 6

1. Schlueter, A.K. and Johnston, C.S., 2011, 'Vitamin C: overview and update', *Journal of Evidence-Based Complementary & Alternative Medicine*, vol. 16, no. 49, pp. 49–55.

2. ibid.

3. Johnston, C.S., et al., 1996, 'Vitamin C depletion is associated with alterations in blood histamine and plasma free carnitine in adults', *Journal of the American College of Nutrition*, vol. 15, pp. 586–91.

4. Clemetson, C.A.B., 2003, 'Elevated blood histamine caused by vaccinations and vitamin C deficiency may mimic the shaken baby syndrome', *Medical Hypothesis*, vol. 62, no. 4, pp. 533–6.

5. Popovich, D., et al., 2009, 'Scurvy forgotten but definitely not gone', *Journal of Pediatric Health Care*, vol. 23, no. 6, pp. 405–15.

6. Schlueter, A.K. and Johnston, C.S., loc. cit.

7. Clemetson, C.A.B., loc. cit.

8. Gundersen, R.Y., et al., 2005, 'Glycine — an important neurotransmitter and cyto-protective agent', *Acta Anaesthesiologica Scandinavica*, vol. 49. no. 8, pp. 1108–16.

9. Booken, D., et al., 2008, 'Glycine receptors are present in human epidermis', *Open Journal of Dermatology*, vol. 2, pp 51–6.

10. ibid.

11. Booken, D., et al., loc. cit.

12. Roth, K.S., 1981, 'Biotin in clinical medicine — a review', *American Journal of Clinical Nutrition*, vol. 34, pp. 1967–74.

13. Baugh, C.M., Malone, J.H. and Butterworth, C.E., 1968, 'Human biotin deficiency', *American Journal of Clinical Nutrition*, vol. 21, pp. 173–182.

14. Sydenstricker, V.P., et al., 1942, 'Observations on the "egg white injury" in man and its cure with a biotin concentrate', *Journal of the American Medical Association*, vol. 118, no. 14, pp. 1199–200.

15. Roth, K.S., loc. cit.

16. ibid.

17. Baugh, C.M., Malone, J.H. and Butterworth, C.E., loc. cit.

18. Mine, Y. and Yang, M., 2008, 'Recent advances in the understanding of egg allergens: basic, industrial, and clinical perspectives', *Journal of Agricultural and Food Chemistry*, vol. 56, pp. 4874–900.

19. Meydani, S.N. et al., 1991, 'Vitamin B6 deficiency impairs interleukin 2 production and lymphocyte proliferation in elderly adults', *American Journal of Clinical Nutrition*, vol. 53, no. 5, pp. 1275–80.

20. Stanton, R., 2007, *Rosemary Stanton's*

Complete Book of Food and Nutrition, Simon & Schuster.

21. Richelle, M., et al., 2006, 'Skin bioavailability of dietary vitamin E, carteniods, polyphenols, vitamin C, zinc and selenium', *British Journal of Nutrition*, vol. 96, pp. 227–38.

22. Anderson, R.A., et al., 1991, 'Supplemental-chromium effects on glucose, insulin, glucagon, and urinary chromium losses in subjects consuming controlled low-chromium diets', *American Journal of Clinical Nutrition*, vol. 54, pp. 909–16.

23. Sidbury, R., et al., 2008, 'Randomised controlled trial of vitamin D supplementation for winter–related atopic dermatitis in Boston: a pilot study', *British Journal of Dermatology*, vol. 159, pp. 245–6.

24. Holick, M.F., 2007, 'Vitamin D deficiency', *New England Journal of Medicine*, vol. 357, no. 3, pp. 266–81.

25. Staberg, B., et al., 1987, 'Abnormal vitamin D metabolism in patients with psoriasis', *Acta Dermato-Venereologica*, vol. 67, no. 1, abstract, retrieved 22 August 2006: http://www.ncbi.nlm.nih.gov/pubmed/2436417./

26. Sidbury, R., et al., loc. cit.

27. Holick, M.F., loc. cit.

28. Sidbury, R., et al., loc. cit.

29. Thiele, J.J. and Ekanayake-Mudiyanselage, S., 2007, 'Vitamin E in human skin: organ-specific physiology and considerations for its use in dermatology', *Molecular Aspects of Medicine*, vol. 28, pp. 646–67.

30. Tsoureli-Nikita, E., Hercogova, J., Lotti, T. and Menchini, G., 2002, 'Evaluation of dietary intake of vitamin E in the treatment of atopic dermatitis: a study of the clinical course and evaluation of the immunoglobulin E serum levels', *International Journal of Dermatology*, vol. 41, no. 3, pp. 146–50.

31. Kahraman, A., et al., 2003, 'The antioxidative and antihistaminic properties of quercetin in ethanol-induced gastric lesions', *Toxicology*, vol. 183, no. 1–3, pp. 133–42.

32. Gupta, C., et al., loc. cit.

33. De Spirt, S. et al., 2009, 'Intervention with flaxseed and borage oil supplements modulates skin condition in women', *British Journal of Nutrition*, vol. 101, pp. 440–45.

34. Boelsma, E., et al., 2003, 'Human skin condition and its associations with nutrient concentrations in serum and diet', *American Journal of Clinical Nutrition*, vol. 77, pp. 348–55.

35. Kalliomäki, M., et al., 2001, 'Probiotics in primary prevention of atopic disease: a randomised placebo-controlled trial', *The Lancet*, vol. 357, pp. 1076–9.

36. Penders, J., et al., loc. cit.

37. Kalliomäki, M., et al., loc. cit.

38. ibid.

39. West, C.E., et al., 2009, 'Probiotics during weaning reduce the incidence of eczema', *Pediatric Allergy and Immunology*, vol. 20, no. 5, pp. 430–7.

40. Ly, N.P., et al., 2011, 'Gut microbiota, probiotics and vitamin D: interrelated exposures influencing allergy, asthma and obesity', *Clinical Reviews in Allergy and Immunology*, vol. 127, pp. 1087–94.

41. Kalliomäki M., et al., 2003, 'Probiotics and prevention of atopic disease: 4-year follow-up of a randomised placebo-controlled trial', *The Lancet*, vol. 361, no. 9372, pp. 1869–71.

42. Hawrelak, J., 2002, 'Probiotics: are supplements really better than yoghurt?' *Journal of the Australian Traditional-Medicine Society*, vol. 8, no. 1, pp. 11–23.

43. Hawrelak, J., 2003, 'Probiotics: choosing the right one for your

needs', *Journal of the Australian Traditional-Medicine Society*, vol. 9, no. 2, pp. 67–75.

44. Rosenfeldt V., et al., 2003, 'Effect of probiotic Lactobacillus strains in children with atopic dermatitis', *Journal of Allergy and Clinical Immunology*, vol. 111, pp. 389–95.

45. Isolauri E., et al., 2000, 'Probiotics in the management of atopic eczema', *Clinical and Experimental Allergy*, vol. 30, pp. 1604–10.

46. Boelsma, E., 2003, loc. cit.

47. ibid.

48. Ehrlich, S.D., 2009, 'Calcium', University of Maryland Medical Centre, retrieved 7 September 2011: www.umm.edu/health/medical/altmed/supplement/calcium./

49. Boelsma, E., 2003, loc. cit.

50. Stanton, R., 2007, loc. cit.

Chapter 8

1. Schor, J., 2010, 'Emotions and health: laughter really is good medicine', *Natural Medicine Journal*, vol. 2, no. 1, pp. 1–4.

2. Kimata, H., 2007, 'Laughter elevates the levels of breastmilk melatonin', *Journal of Psychosomatic Research*, vol. 62, no. 6, pp. 699–702.

3. Olesen, A.B., et al., 2003, 'Atopic dermatitis is increased following vaccination for measles, mumps and rubella or measles infection', *Acta Dermato-Venereologica*, vol. 83, pp. 445–50.

4. Pickering L.K. (ed.), 2003, *Red Book: 2003 Report of the Committee on Infectious Diseases*, 26th edition, Elk Grove Village, Ill: American Academy of Pediatrics.

Chapter 10

1. Dawson, T.L., 2007, '*Malassezia globosa and restricta*: breakthrough understanding of the etiology and treatment of dandruff and seborrheic dermatitis through whole-genome analysis', *Journal of Investigative Dermatology Symposium Proceedings*, vol. 12, pp. 15–9.

2. ibid.

3. McGinley, K.J., et al., 1975, 'Quantitative microbiology of the scalp in non-dandruff and seborrheic dermatitis', *Journal of Investigative Dermatology*, vol. 64, no. 6, pp. 401–5.

4. ibid.

Chapter 13

1. Sariachvili, M., et al., 2010, 'Early exposure to solid foods and the development of eczema in children up to 4 years of age', *Pediatric Allergy and Immunology*, vol. 21, no. 1 (part 1), pp. 74–81.

Chapter 17

1. Kelble, A., 2005, 'Spices and type 2 diabetes', *Nutrition and Food Science*, vol. 35, no. 2, pp. 81–7.

Index